PEDIATRIC EDUCATION AND THE NEEDS OF EXCEPTIONAL CHILDREN

PEDIATRIC EDUCATION AND THE NEEDS OF EXCEPTIONAL CHILDREN

edited by

Michael J. Guralnick, Ph.D.
Director, The Nisonger Center
Professor of Communication and Psychology,
The Ohio State University

and

H. Burtt Richardson, Jr., M.D.
Adjunct Associate Professor of
Child Health and Development,
George Washington University School of Medicine
and Health Sciences
Pediatrician, Winthrop Area Medical Center,
Winthrop, Maine

University Park Press
Baltimore

UNIVERSITY PARK PRESS
International Publishers in Science, Medicine, and Education
233 East Redwood Street
Baltimore, Maryland 21202

Composed by University Park Press, Typesetting Division
Manufactured in the United States of America by The Maple Press Company

Library of Congress Cataloging in Publication Data
Main entry under title:
Pediatric education and the needs of exceptional children.
Based on a conference held in June, 1978 at Children's Hospital National
Medical Center, Washington, D.C.
Bibliography: p.
Includes index.
1. Pediatrics—Study and teaching—Congresses. 2. Exceptional children—Care
and treatment—Study and teaching—Congresses. 3. Handicapped children—
Care and treatment—Study and teaching—Congresses. 4. Child development—
Study and teaching—Congress. I. Guralnick, Michael J. II. Richardson, Henry
Burtt, 1934-   [DNLM: 1. Education of mentally retarded. LC4661 P371]
RJ80.P4   618.9'2   79-9167
ISBN 0-8391-1500-8

Contents

Contributors

Pasquale J. Accardo, M.D.
Developmental Pediatrician, John F.
Kennedy Institute
Assistant Professor of Pediatrics
Johns Hopkins University School
of Medicine
Baltimore, Maryland 21205

Nicholas J. Anastasiow, Ph.D.
Associate Director for Research
John F. Kennedy Child Development
Center
University of Colorado Health
Sciences Center
Denver, Colorado 80262

John B. Bartram, M.D.*
Handicapped Children's Unit
St. Christopher's Hospital for
Children
Professor Emeritus of Pediatrics
Temple University School of
Medicine
Philadelphia, Pennsylvania 19133

Forrest C. Bennett, M.D.*
Director of Medical Education,
Clinical Training Unit/CDMRC
Assistant Professor of Pediatrics
University of Washington
Seattle, Washington 98195

T. Berry Brazelton, M.D.*
Chief, Child Development Unit
Children's Hospital Medical Center
Associate Professor of Pediatrics
Harvard Medical School
Boston, Massachusetts 02115

Arnold J. Capute, M.D., M.P.H.*
Deputy Director and Director of
Clinical Services
John F. Kennedy Institute
Associate Professor of Pediatrics
Johns Hopkins University School of
Medicine
Baltimore, Maryland 21205

Marlin E. Cohrs
Media Director
John F. Kennedy Child Develop-
ment Center
University of Colorado Health
Sciences Center
Denver, Colorado 80262

Stephen C. Copps, M.D.*
Director, Western Wisconsin Neuro-
development Evaluation and
Treatment Center
Gundersen Clinic
La Crosse, Wisconsin 54601

Donald W. Delaney, M.D.*
Associate Director for Patient Care
and Educational Coordination
Children's Hospital National Medical
Center
Professor and Associate Chairman
of Child Health and Development
George Washington University School
of Medicine and Health Sciences
Washington, D.C. 20010

---

*Indicates conference participant

William K. Frankenburg, M.D.*
Director
John F. Kennedy Child Development
  Center
Professor of Pediatrics and Preventive Medicine
University of Colorado Health
  Sciences Center
Denver, Colorado 80262

Marvin I. Gottlieb, M.D., Ph.D.*
Chief, Section of Developmental and
  Behavioral Pediatrics
Professor of Pediatrics
University of Tennessee Center for
  the Health Sciences
Memphis, Tennessee 38163

Michael J. Guralnick, Ph.D.*
Director, The Nisonger Center
Professor of Communication and
  Psychology
The Ohio State University
Columbus, Ohio 43210

Vince L. Hutchins, M.D.*
Associate Director, Bureau of Community Health Services
Office for Maternal and Child
  Health
Department of Health, Education and
  Welfare
Rockville, Maryland 20857

Douglas R. Kutner, Ph.D.
Research Associate, The Nisonger
  Center
The Ohio State University
Columbus, Ohio 43210

Melvin D. Levine, M.D.
Chief, Division of Ambulatory
  Pediatrics
Children's Hospital Medical Center
Assistant Professor of Pediatrics
Harvard University School of
  Medicine
Boston, Massachusetts 02115

Michael S. Levine, M.D.
Pediatrician, Curative Rehabilitation
  Center
Assistant Professor of Pediatrics and
  Physical Medicine and Rehabilitation

Medical College of Wisconsin
Milwaukee, Wisconsin 53226

Gerhard E. Martin, M.D.
Chief of Neurology, The Nisonger
  Center
Adjunct Associate Professor of
  Neurology
The Ohio State University
Columbus, Ohio 43210

Richard W. Olmsted, M.D.*
Medical Director, Children's Hospital
Professor of Pediatrics
University of Colorado Medical
  Center
Denver, Colorado 80218

H. Burtt Richardson, Jr., M.D.*
Adjunct Associate Professor of Child
  Health and Development
George Washington University School
  of Medicine and Health Sciences
Washington, D.C.
Pediatrician, Winthrop Area Medical
  Center
Winthrop, Maine 04364

William Sammons, M.D.,
Fellow, Child Development Unit
Children's Hospital Medical Center
Fellow in Medicine (Child Development)
Harvard Medical School
Boston, Massachusetts 02115

Arthur H. Stengel, M. A.
Research Associate, Institute for
  Child Study
Indiana University
Bloomington, Indiana 47401

William W. Swan, Ed.D.*
Acting Chief, Early Childhood
  Section
Bureau of Education for the Handicapped
Office of Education
Department of Health, Education and
  Welfare
Washington, D.C. 20202

Lawrence T. Taft, M.D.
Professor and Chairman, Department
  of Pediatrics
Rutgers Medical School
New Jersey College of Medicine and
  Dentistry
Piscataway, New Jersey 08854

Victor C. Vaughan, III, M.D.*
Professor of Pediatrics
Temple University School of Medicine
Senior Fellow in Medical Evaluation
National Board of Medical Examiners
Philadelphia, Pennsylvania 19104

Michael W. Yogman, M.D.*
Associate in Medicine
Children's Hospital Medical Center
Instructor in Pediatrics
Harvard Medical School
Boston, Massachusetts 02115

Peter W. Zinkus, Ph.D.*
Assistant Professor of Pediatrics
Section of Developmental and
  Behavioral Pediatrics
University of Tennessee Center for
  the Health Sciences
Memphis, Tennessee 38163

Mark L. Wolraich, M.D.*
Director of Pediatric Education
Division of Developmental Disabilities
Assistant Professor of Pediatrics
University of Iowa
Iowa City, Iowa 52242

Preface

The conference upon which this book is based, Pediatric Education and the Needs of Young Exceptional Children, brought together pediatric educators prominent in teaching about exceptional children to medical students, residents, fellows, and practicing pediatricians. Conference presentations provided background perspectives and current examples of educational curricula to assist each pediatric department or training program to establish or modify, where appropriate, this aspect of pediatric education. Building upon the conference, however, and recognizing the clear need ultimately to develop a comprehensive, generally accepted, focused, and carefully validated curriculum, we expanded this volume beyond the conference presentations to include additional material. This permitted us to attempt to establish a firm rationale and to provide a conceptual and organizational framework for the future design, implementation, and evaluation of a curriculum that would enable physicians to meet effectively the needs of exceptional children and their families.

We attempted to address issues that were critical from a broad educational perspective, including considerations of curriculum design, methodology, implementation strategies, and evaluation technology. Matters of content were also discussed, but mostly at the level of identifying significant educational goals and objectives. Major content areas that appeared with great frequency included training issues related to long-term management, the nature of interdisciplinary involvement, essential knowledge in child development, the varied and changing role of the pediatrician, and sensitivity to the complex problems of exceptional children and their families.

The book is divided into three main sections. The first, focusing on background and rationale, consists of seven chapters and is designed to set the stage for the more detailed program descriptions that follow. In the first chapter, Guralnick, Richardson, and Kutner examine pediatric education in relation to the development of exceptional children. The role of pediatricians, management and interdisciplinary issues, parent perspectives, and interactions with special educators are discussed. In addition, a critical review of related training programs is presented and discussed in terms of the recent report by The Task Force on Pediatric Education.

Major legislation and programs affecting handicapped children have been enacted in recent years. Hutchins and Swan, in the second chapter, highlight these critical developments from a federal perspective and relate them to physician involvement and associated funding issues. Following this, two chapters are presented to emphasize the educational implications of recent child development concepts, physician-family relationships, and parental processes of adaptation. In the first, Anastasiow and Stengel describe the value of a transactional approach to development with special emphasis on the need to assess the child's ecology, particularly the socialization practices of parents. Yogman, Sammons, and Brazelton then focus on the adaptations of both families and physicians, the timing and form of clinical intervention, and how this information might be incorporated into the medical school curriculum.

Systematic approaches to curriculum design and evaluation are presented in the next chapters. M. S. Levine emphasizes the need for establishing a unified conceptual framework and outlines the hierarchical and sequential relationships among curricular elements. In Vaughan's chapter an emphasis is placed on organizing and evaluating the competencies of pediatricians. In doing so, he presents a thorough analysis of the tasks-by-abilities matrix and its potential application to the area of exceptional children. As will be noted, a number of training programs described in the second section of this book have utilized versions of this model.

In the final chapter of the first section, Delaney, Bartram, Olmsted, and Copps provide an overview of educational objectives and strategies as well as barriers to implementation at the various training levels.

The second section of the book is devoted to descriptions of current programs at the medical student, residency, fellowship, and continuing education levels. Gottlieb and Zinkus present a medical student curriculum and make a particularly valuable distinction between the private practice-oriented model and the academically-oriented model.

The three chapters that follow focus on residency programs. First, Wolraich describes a curriculum for a 1-month rotation in developmental disabilities as well as the results of his efforts to document program effectiveness. The chapter by Bennett describes the activities of residents involved in an unusually extensive 3-month residency rotation in child development and handicapping conditions. The positive evaluation of this training program, as accomplished through resident feedback relative to clinical experience, questionnaires to practicing pediatricians following completion of the program, and Board scores in comparison to national norms, was particularly valuable. This emphasis on the importance of evaluation and accountability is further amplified in work by Richardson and Guralnick. In this chapter an evaluation strategy compatible with the practical constraints inherent in pediatric rotations but containing a high degree of objectivity and internal validity is presented.

The chapter by Capute and Accardo describes a multi-year fellowship program in developmental pediatrics. Their description of the inpatient and outpatient rotations and the variety of specialty rotations offered provide a comprehensive picture of such a fellowship training program. These authors also emphasize that a truly adequate fellowship experience must build upon developmental principles that have been introduced at all levels of medical training.

The development of training strategies for practicing pediatricians poses unique problems, such as geographic and time constraints. In their chapter, Frankenburg and Cohrs address these issues and present a well-developed model for providing short-term training to practitioners in developmental diagnosis. Zinkus and Gottlieb are also concerned with these problems and describe such strategies as intensive study programs and mini-residencies for practicing pediatricians in their chapter.

In the final chapter of this section Martin focuses on the role of the pediatric neurologist in the management of developmental disabilities. Of special interest is his discussion of the interrelationships between pediatric residency curricula in developmental disabilities and residency programs for pediatric neurologists.

The last section of the book, "Framework for Future Efforts," consists of a chapter by Richardson, Guralnick, Taft, and M. D. Levine that attempts to summarize and integrate the essential characteristics of a curriculum in child development and handicapping conditions in terms of its design, implementation, and evaluation components. Drawing upon many sources, twelve goals and examples of specific content are identified along with specific suggestions for curriculum design and implementation strategies. Finally, an example of a clinical problem based on this outline of a comprehensive curriculum is cast into the tasks-by-abilities matrix as a means for evaluation.

The conference was held in Washington, D.C. at Children's Hospital National Medical Center in June, 1978. Dr. Robert H. Parrott, director of the hospital, provided facilities for the conference and his support is gratefully acknowledged. Funding for the conference was provided primarily by the U.S. Office of Education's Bureau of Education for the Handicapped, Program Development Branch, through the Handicapped Children's Early Education Program. It has been through this agency's continuing support of our efforts that we have been able to follow through on the linkage between pediatric education and the needs of exceptional children.

Joint sponsorship of the conference was provided by Children's Hospital National Medical Center and the Department of Child Health and Development of the George Washington University School of Medicine, Washington, D.C.; the National Children's Center, Washington, D.C.; and The Nisonger Center, The Ohio State University. Special thanks are due to the staff of the National Children's Center, especially Deborah Tupper.

Editing a volume such as this is always the product of many individuals. Outstanding in this regard was the work of Ellen Weinhouse for critically reviewing the manuscript. Most significant, however, were the contributions of Marilee Darr. Her technical editing skills and keen sense of organization were major factors in the successful completion of this book.

Finally, we wish to thank the contributors to this volume for sharing their ideas, enthusiasm, programs, and aspirations. We are hopeful that their efforts will stimulate both the thinking and actions of those concerned with pediatric education and exceptional children.

PEDIATRIC EDUCATION AND THE NEEDS OF EXCEPTIONAL CHILDREN

section I

BACKGROUND AND RATIONALE

chapter 1

PEDIATRIC EDUCATION AND THE DEVELOPMENT OF EXCEPTIONAL CHILDREN

Michael J. Guralnick, H. Burtt Richardson, Jr., and Douglas R. Kutner

The passage of the Education for All Handicapped Children Act of 1975, Public Law 94-142, is a landmark in a continuing evolutionary process affirming and reaffirming the rights, privileges, and responsibilities of handicapped individuals. The enactment of this law, focusing primarily on the educational aspects of handicapped children, has been paralleled by similar changes in a variety of other domains, particularly those related to the handicapped individual's right to community living, treatment, and pursuit of a meaningful vocation (Begab and Richardson, 1975; President's Committee on Mental Retardation, 1977). Given the interrelatedness of events at the biological, psychological, social, and economic levels that are associated with virtually every aspect of handicapping conditions, there are few professional groups that are unaffected by these changes. Although the implications of this process of social change will certainly vary from group to group, it is clear that some form of modification in attitudes, knowledge, and technical and clinical skills are likely to be essential in order to optimize the developmental opportunities of handicapped children.

A major focus of this chapter is to explore the relationship between the education of pediatricians and the needs of exceptional children

Portions of this chapter were supported by Grant OEG-0-77-00705 from the U.S. Office of Education, Bureau of Education for the Handicapped.

within the framework of these social developments. In doing so, this chapter first identifies the basis for recommending the expansion and modification of training programs in handicapping conditions for pediatricians. Data from various surveys of pediatricians, pediatric educators, and parents are organized and analyzed and linked to the nature of the responsibilities that pediatricians are expected to assume. Subsequently, a wide range of training programs are reviewed and evaluated to assist in forming conclusions about the state-of-the-art and the projected training needs.

OVERVIEW OF THE ROLE OF THE
PEDIATRICIAN: IMPLICATIONS FOR TRAINING

Increased Involvement by Pediatricians

Analyzing an earlier survey on the adequacy of pediatric residency programs by the Joint Committee on Pediatric Research, Education, and Practice (PREP) (see Cooke, 1966), de la Cruz (1976) asked the following question: "In light of the changing pattern of pediatric care, which has resulted in an increasing involvement of pediatricians in the emotional, social, and learning problems of children, are pediatricians properly trained to meet this need?" (p. 689). Unfortunately, his answer to that question was that significant training needs do exist. For example, the PREP survey revealed that although 60% of the practicing pediatricians who responded indicated that they frequently were involved in the management of mental and emotional disorders, 35% felt that they had low competence in dealing with these problems. Moreover, 57% of the practitioners reported that, during residency, training opportunities for continuing care of various manifestations of "chronic cerebral dysfunction" were insufficient.

The perceived lack of competence and the need for more extensive training probably reflect, in part, the practitioner's recognition of the extraordinary complexity of problems associated with handicapped individuals. Specifically, individuals with handicapping conditions have difficulties that are multidimensional, that range over many levels, that are generally accompanied by significant family stress, and that have broad social and economic implications. One outcome of this state of affairs is the multiplicity of roles, particularly with regard to coordination, that is often thrust upon one key professional — frequently, the primary physician — by the families of handicapped individuals. The role of pediatricians in this regard, especially in relation to management on a long-range basis, is explored in the next section.

Coordination, Management, and the Interdisciplinary Team

As discussed by Battle (1972), the team approach is a necessity when dealing with the problems of chronic handicapping conditions, but she clearly recognizes the difficulties that are associated with integrating the team's findings. Battle suggests that a leadership role, analogous to the role of an ombudsman, be adopted by the pediatrician, who organizes the treatment program based upon a total perspective of the problem and utilizes other specialists, but who is the prime interpreter for the parents. Referring to this coordinating role, Battle states:

> This should not prevent their [the parents'] direct contact with the specialist, which they need and have the right to expect. Rather, the pediatrician's role is to help the family in a situation which may be overwhelming if they are bombarded with a list of recommendations from a multitude of specialists. It is his role to shape the recommendations of the various disciplines into a long-range program (p. 922).

It is also important to note that the adoption of this role by the physician, going well beyond general medical care, is supported in the field by many individuals (see Solomons and Menolascino, 1968; Johnston, 1976) and organizations (e.g., see the American Academy of Pediatrics Committee on Children with Handicaps' publication, *The Pediatrician and the Child with Mental Retardation* [Koch and Kugel, 1971]).

Despite the many sound arguments that logically point to this role (especially the fact that the physician is, in many instances, most likely to be in a position to ensure continuity of care for the young handicapped child), we can expect the pediatrician to play numerous roles, ranging from a significant coordinating role to one of a consultant. The adoption of these roles may occur either formally, through designation by interdisciplinary teams, or informally, as part of the normal physician-patient relationship. Such a determination will vary with individual circumstances, but depends upon the nature of client needs and the availability of services, especially trained professionals in other disciplines.

Related to the physician's role is the concept of long-term management. Since effective coordination of the interdisciplinary process extends beyond diagnostic and evaluation procedures to the ability to manage the complexities of the problems of exceptional children, the designation of roles must consider this fact. Unfortunately, it is precisely this management role that appears to be lacking in the training of pediatricians. As Pearson (1968) points out: "Mental retardation is the major handicapping condition in childhood, yet many physicians, including pediatricians, are unfamiliar with their role in management" (p. 835).

The Interdisciplinary Process

It is frustrating to note that although the interdisciplinary team process appears essential for effective evaluation and treatment planning for children with chronic disabilities, group problem-solving in this form is one of the most difficult processes to carry out successfully. Johnston and Magrab (1976) point out that the dynamics of a team's functioning must be recognized, and that this recognition often requires considerable interpersonal skills. For example, they note that the emotional climate, particularly such factors as trust, openness, respect, and interdependence, must be favorable for effective decision-making to occur.

The concept of interdisciplinary training is the focal point of activities related to University Affiliated Facilities (UAFs). It is worthwhile here to present the definition of interdisciplinary training accepted by the UAF training program directors:

> Interdisciplinary training is an integrated educational process involving the interdependent contributions of the several relevant disciplines designed to enhance professional growth as it relates to training, service, and research. The interdisciplinary process promotes the development and use of a basic language, a core body of knowledge, relevant skills, and an understanding of the attitude, values, and method of participating disciplines (Tarjan, 1976, p. 11).

Involvement of pediatricians in training programs designed to promote relevant knowledge, skills, attitudes, and values is critical to the interdisciplinary process.

Parent Perspectives

Parents have probably been the most vocal group in expressing their dissatisfaction with regard to the pediatrician's skills, sensitivity, and knowledge in managing children with chronic disabilities. The feelings of many parents, based upon an extensive parent survey, are perhaps best summarized by the following statement:

> When [the physician] is confronted by a patient whom he cannot cure as one cures an infection, a disease, a broken limb — by a patient whose problem is chronic and whose rehabilitation, if possible at all, is a matter of years of special education and training — it is, in a very real sense, bad news for him too. He must convey a diagnosis indicating a long-term problem or set of problems, and he will have to deal with the distress it will inevitably provoke. Chances are that his experience with emotionally, mentally, or even physically handicapped children is not great. His training in medical school to handle such children and their parents was probably slight. He is a professional, but he is also human, and rather understandably uncomfortable with the situation. He may seek refuge from his discomfort by pronouncing his diagnosis and terminating his responsibility for and involvement with the patient as best he can — by referring the child to someone else or, if the seriousness of

the disability seems to him to warrant it, by recommending that the child be institutionalized. Sometimes he may state his diagnosis and interpret it to the parents, but be unable to tell them where to go for the nonmedical services which are the next step for his patient. He is there to cure sick children, and this is not a sick child. He is a busy man and may feel that he simply cannot be responsible for knowing the realm of specialized non-medical services available for handicapped children (Gorham et al., 1975, p. 157).

If these observations are accurate, extensive educational efforts are in order. This is particularly true in light of the last comment by Gorham et al., because without an awareness of community resources and a willingness to make recommendations to relevant professionals and organizations, the coordinating role is not possible.

Unfortunately, the investigation of Kelly and Menolascino (1975) into physicians' awareness of community-based services and attitudes toward mentally retarded individuals tends to support the fact that such knowledge and positive attitudes are held by only a small fraction of physicians. Surveying physicians in a midwestern city offering extensive and varied alternative programs to retarded individuals, Kelly and Menolascino found that a substantial proportion of physicians were not familiar with some of the major service agencies. In fact, there was a large discrepancy between the reports by physicians with regard to their perception of their counseling and advising of parents and the counseling that was perceived by the parents. For example, 71% of the physicians indicated that they provided materials about retardation to parents, but only 10% of the parents said that they received them. Apparently, serious communication gaps exist. In addition, this study highlighted the fact that although parents were generally satisfied with medical advice and treatment, 57% were dissatisfied with the physician's "attitude" toward their retarded child. One final note is that despite the fact that physicians had only a limited awareness of the range of community alternatives, virtually all those surveyed felt that it was their responsibility to recommend institutionalization.

Interviewing and Counseling

Professionals are keenly aware of the importance of counseling parents of handicapped children in an effective manner (see Begab, 1971; Farber, 1975). Solomons and Menolascino (1968) have stressed the critical nature of the initial interview by the primary physician and have provided guidelines for the subsequent counseling of parents (see Chapter 4, this volume). In particular, they emphasize the interpersonal aspects of the interview and counseling process, yet it is precisely these characteristics that parents complain are frequently lacking. A partial explanation for this can perhaps be found in the report by Helfer (1970) on pediatric interviewing skills. Analyzing videotapes of simulated interviews of mothers of children with serious organic illnesses and related psychosocia problems, a number of significant differences emerged through comparisons of freshmen and senior medical students. Of most relevance to this discussion was the finding that although seniors obtained more factual information related to organic factors, they obtained less interpersonal information and asked fewer open-ended questions. In general, the interviewing techniques of the seniors appeared quite mechanical and limited to the immediate medical problems; not at all like the skills professionals recommend that are necessary to assist the family. Helfer provides the following example characterizing the differences between the two levels of medical students:

> One programmed mother had a 3-year-old retarded child with meningomyelocele and hydrocephalus. She was 3 months pregnant and most concerned about the outcome of this pregnancy. No senior discovered this fact in his interview. The first freshman who interviewed her asked, "Are you going to have any more children?" After learning of her pregnancy he replied, "You must be worried that you'll have another baby with the same problem?" (pp. 625–626).

REVIEW OF TRAINING PROGRAMS

With this background, it is important to examine the extent and nature of training programs that have been implemented for medical students and residents that relate to exceptional children and their families. Such an analysis may help us understand some of the concerns expressed in this chapter, as well as identify directions for change. Furthermore, this chapter focuses on the results of published programs or surveys. (Section two of this book presents additional programs.)

Oster (1974) has provided us with an excellent historical review of training programs in mental retardation for medical students. He noted that Bradley's (1953) work at the University of Oregon appeared to be the first documented program. Frequently, the pattern of training was based on an affiliation between mental retardation training centers and institutions, such as the relationship between Yale Medical School and the Southbury Training School. For the most part, the programs that Oster was able to identify were of an informal nature, consisting of overall descriptions of training opportunities with little in the way of systematic educational experiences or the evaluation of the student's experience.

Surveys

Oster (1974) also reported on a survey of medical schools in which faculty, students, and recent graduates in various countries were surveyed in an effort to determine the nature of the educational experiences in mental retardation and other handicapping conditions that the students had obtained. His review and findings generally provided a very pessimistic picture of the state of the art as summarized in the following statement:

> Taking everything into consideration, it may be stated that apparently few hours are employed to deal with [both mental retardation and other handicapping conditions] round about in the world. These hours are very few indeed when it is considered that a considerable percentage of the clientele of the general practitioner are involved in these problems. Many university lecturers express regret about this and explain and excuse it by the fact that their curriculum is already particularly limited. Nevertheless, this need not prevent alterations and possibly improvements in the teaching programmes within the same limited time, as some have suggested. One thing stands out very clearly, that communication between disciplines shows catastrophic deficiencies and coordination between teaching programmes is only present in a very few centres where these fields are concerned.
>
> The majority of teachers consider that teaching in their own particular discipline is organized or even well-planned. This shows a great contrast with the opinions of the recently qualified doctors, none of whom shared the opinion of their teachers. They had all recently come from the teaching they received as students and they felt that the teaching they had received concerning [mental retardation] was scattered, haphazard and without coordination or plan (p. 26).

More recent information can be found in Pilkington's (1977) survey of all the medical schools in the United Kingdom and Ireland. This study essentially supported earlier findings that stated that educational programs in handicapping conditions for medical students were fragmented and that no true interdisciplinary program existed. Moreover, the recently published (1978) Task Force report on pediatric education (reviewed in detail below) further documented and reinforced the need for improved pediatric education programs in this area.

Evaluation and Content of Specific Programs

When evaluation has been utilized at all, it has generally consisted of pretest/posttest assessments. For example, Fishler et al., (1968) assessed the effect of a 3-week clerkship in a Child Development Clinic on medical students' responses to a questionnaire designed to reflect various attitudes toward mental retardation. The clerkship consisted of observation of and participation with a multidisciplinary diagnostic evaluation team, which included diagnosis, assessment, staffings, and parent counseling. Although the program had some positive impact, the most revealing finding indicated by the pretest was the fact that even fourth year medical students showed very little recognition of the broad social implications of mental retardation, or of the physician's role in the counseling of parents of retarded children.

More recently, Simeonsson, Kenny, and Walker (1976) developed and evaluated a training program for fourth year medical students participating in a 1-month rotation through a pediatric diagnostic clinic for developmentally disabled children. Using a pretest/posttest design measuring both knowledge (through objective questions) and attitudes (through an attitude scale), this program had a significant effect on the medical students' attitudes. These results, in conjunction with the Fishler et al. (1968) findings, suggest the strong need for positive training experiences in handicapping conditions for medical students.

At the residency level, Richardson, Guralnick, and Tupper (1978) developed a program focusing on the following 11 objectives:

> 1) gain sensitivity to and comfort with individual handicapped children (Children), 2) gain awareness of the behavioral characteristics of different handicapped children (Behavior), 3) gain familiarity with labels and other terminology used to describe handicapped children (Labels), 4) gain understanding of the limits of labeling (Limits), 5) gain knowledge of the terminology of special education (Special Education), 6) gain knowledge of tests used to evaluate handicapped children (Tests), 7) gain knowledge of psychological terminology and the role of psychologists in the management of handicapped children (Psychologist), 8) gain knowledge of social work terminology and the role of the social worker (Social Worker), 9) gain ability to communicate effectively and plan with parents concerning the developmental and educational needs of a handicapped child (Parents), 10) gain ability to communicate effectively with teachers about the developmental and educational needs of a handicapped child (Teachers), and 11) gain understanding of community resources available for handicapped children (Community) (p. 4).

At the outset, the major interest of this investigation was assessing the residents' judgments of the importance of these objectives as part of their training, as well as determining the feasibility of the training program. Accordingly, following training, residents rated each of the 11 objectives on a 9-point scale. (The midpoint of the scale was 5 indicating "possibly important or effective.") Figure 1 indicates that all objectives were considered to be important, particularly those related to parents and teachers. As can be seen, the program's effectiveness in carrying out these objectives varied somewhat, with objectives related to teachers, community resources, behavior, and limits appearing to be more effectively carried out.

Another perspective was obtained by asking the residents to appraise subjectively their progress from the beginning to the end of training in terms of their "competence and confidence" with regard to each of the program's objectives. Figure 2 reveals that residents perceived that progress occurred for all objectives, but particularly in relation to community resources. A more systematic and objective evaluation of this short-term curriculum (12 hours direct contact time across a 4-week period) was also

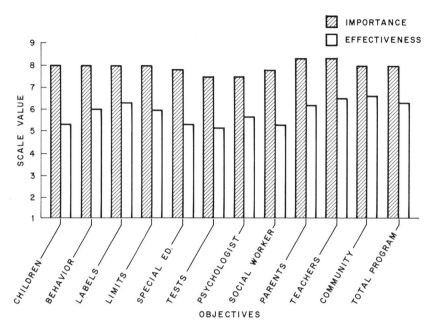

Figure 1.   Ratings by pediatric residents of the importance and effectiveness for each of the program's objectives. (Reprinted by permission from Richardson, Guralnick, and Tupper, 1978.)

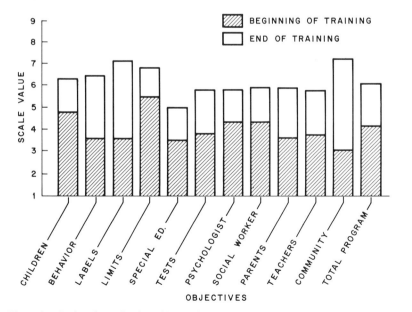

Figure 2.   Ratings by pediatric residents of their competence and confidence for each of the program's objectives at the beginning and end of training. (Reprinted by permission from Richardson, Guralnick, and Tupper, 1978.)

carried out and is summarized by Richardson and Guralnick. (See Chapter 11, this volume, and Richardson and Guralnick, 1978.)

It is important to note that training activities were conducted and integrated with a preschool program for handicapped children. The program permitted the residents to obtain a very different perspective from the perspective that develops in programs where training activities are related to a diagnostic and evaluation clinic. In particular, the focus on the management aspects of problems — the clear link with special educators and the other professionals who are involved with the child and the perspective gained from seeing children over time in a social setting — were suggested by the residents as being highly positive characteristics of the training program.

Implications

This review of the published literature on training programs concerned with handicapped children and their families at the various levels of training has revealed at least two consistent patterns. First, virtually all programs could be characterized as "preliminary." Very rarely were programs well developed, nor had they been subjected to revisions based on repeated evaluations and feedback. Second, each program seemed independent of all other programs. Although a variety of professional organizations were and are potentially available to help coordinate the development and implementation of programs, no such efforts were apparent.

**TASK FORCE REPORT ON PEDIATRIC
EDUCATION IN RELATION TO EXCEPTIONAL CHILDREN**

The recent report by The Task Force on Pediatric Education (1978) contains sections relevant to exceptional children and provides the most up-to-date source with regard to perceptions of their educational needs by pediatricians in this area. The report consists of both the impressions gleaned from 2 years of intensive deliberations involving numerous groups, as well as a description of an extensive survey, and the interpretations of the results.

Of prime importance, the report indicated that the trend toward increased involvement of pediatricians in virtually all aspects of child health and development observed over the past decade, particularly with respect to the management aspects, was still very prominent. The report states:

> Pediatricians will be called upon increasingly to manage children with emotional disturbances, learning disabilities, chronic illnesses, and other problems of a developmental, psychological, and social nature. They will provide increased amounts of health care to adolescents. They will be expected to

manage their practices efficiently, collaborate with other members of the health care team, and utilize community resources to enhance the effectiveness of services to children and their families (p. 13).

With regard to residency training, the report identified a number of underemphasized areas from their survey of over 7,000 recent graduates of pediatric residency programs. Included in that list were the developmental aspects of pediatrics, community pediatrics, and handicapping and chronic conditions.

Table 1 presents data from one major question of the survey concerned with the residency experience that relates most closely to various aspects of exceptional children. Note that nearly 54% of the respondents rated their residency experience with respect to psychosocial and/or behavioral problems as being insufficient. Similar ratings of insufficient experience were noted for manifestations of chronic cerebral dysfunction (40.4%) and interviewing and counseling skills (40.8%). From earlier discussions, it is likely that this latter figure reflects a major contribution from problems encountered in interviewing and counseling parents of exceptional children.

The Task Force survey also revealed that 53% of the respondents rated their competence as low or somewhat low in the area of genetic counseling, and 44.5% rated their residency training as insufficient in this area of practice. Of perhaps most relevance, the survey indicated that 36.3% rated their residency experience as insufficient with respect to managing disorders of mental or emotional development, with nearly the same percentage judging themselves as having a low or somewhat low competence level. Finally, responses to questions in the area of practice labeled neurology and learning disabilities also suggested insufficiencies in residency training with 37.1% of the respondents so indicating.

For community pediatrics, the Task Force summarized the questionnaire results as follows:

Over half the respondents felt they had been insufficiently prepared for involvement in child advocacy (e.g., problems of minority groups, child abuse and neglect, and children with mental retardation), over 60 percent felt inadequately prepared to deal with school health problems, and almost three-fourths felt insufficiently trained in community programs relating to child health and welfare such as custodial institutions, nursery schools, juvenile courts, and programs for exceptional children (pp. 23–24).

It should be noted that comparisons between this survey and the 1965 PREP report indicated improvements in the areas of genetic counseling, neurology, and learning.

Finally, the Task Force report reaffirmed the coordinating, management, and counseling roles that are often assumed by pediatricians. The report states:

Table 1. A question from the Task Force Survey on Pediatric Education concerned with the residency experience

Question Please evaluate your participatory experience in each of the following areas during pediatric residency

	My experience in residency was:			
	Insufficient	Sufficient	Excessive	DK/NA
a. Longitudinal care of well children as opposed to episodic care	50.4%	48.4%	0.5%	0.6%
b. Care of adolescents	65.9%	33.0%	0.3%	0.8%
c. Care of patients with				
1. Chronic diseases such as diabetes, cystic fibrosis, rheumatoid arthritis	18.4%	74.2%	7.0%	0.6%
2. Various manifestations of chronic cerebral dysfunction	40.4%	56.8%	2.1%	0.6%
3. Psychosocial and/or behavioral problems	53.9%	44.1%	1.2%	0.8%
d. Interviewing and counseling	40.8%	57.1%	1.3%	0.8%
e. Ambulatory care				
1. Within the medical school hospital	11.4%	79.9%	7.1%	1.6%
2. Extramural	44.8%	49.6%	1.9%	3.7%

From The Task Force Survey on Pediatric Education. 1978. *The Future of Pediatric Education*. Evanston, Ill.: American Academy of Pediatrics. Reprinted by permission.

The care of the child with a handicap is usually multidisciplinary and on-going, and the role of the pediatrician is normally that of a coordinator of services. Residents should appreciate the role of other disciplines in the care of the disabled child and develop the ability to work cooperatively with them. They should learn to help parents to understand the need for multiple services and the importance of complying with the multitude of recommendations that may be made. A child's disability may place great emotional and financial strain on the parents and other family members. The resident must anticipate such problems and be capable of managing them. The resident must learn to assist the family in marshalling the community resources for the benefit of children with handicapping conditions (pp. 24–25).

Taken together, the Task Force report clearly supports earlier indications that substantial needs remain with regard to pediatric education and exceptional children. In fact, given the increasing involvement of pediatricians in this area, training programs must move rapidly to ensure that the gap between needs and training opportunities does not widen. Finally, the report identified more specifically those areas to which a training curriculum should attend and that can serve as a useful database for curricular design.

PEDIATRICS AND SPECIAL EDUCATION

Revisions and expansions of training programs for pediatricians will likely place considerable emphasis on the relationship with special educators. This is primarily due to the enactment of PL 94-142 which, in part, mandates a free public education, the right to an appropriate education as expressed in the design of individualized educational plans (IEPs), and the right of due process and parent involvement. Moreover, special education must be provided in the least restrictive environment and efforts must be designed to ensure that all handicapped children are identified, located, and evaluated.

In actuality, the responsibilities of pediatricians and other physicians are not identified in PL 94-142. Nevertheless, effective implementation implies essential physician responsibilities in the identification, the evaluation, and the provision of services (Jacobs and Walker, 1978; Palfrey, Mervis, and Butler, 1978). With regard to the design of IEPs, involvement of physicians in these plans represents a potentially important step in the interdisciplinary process. Since these plans emphasize the functional and management aspects of the special educational program, there is a press for all participants to develop practical assessment instruments and recommendations that can lead to meaningful instructional and therapeutic strategies. Analyzed from a broad perspective, full implementation of PL 94-142 implies even further involvement of pediatricians and other physicians in the diagnosis, assessment, evaluation, and management of the handicapped child. Associated with this involvement is the need for additional training, particularly since physician-educator relationships appear to be strained by role expectancy and communications problems (Beck et al., 1978).

The projected strengthening of the relationship between medicine and special education also reflects recognition of the fact that educational settings and educational personnel can significantly contribute to training programs concerned with handicapping conditions for pediatricians. In our opinion, effective participation as a member of a team by any professional requires extensive, direct, and systematic involvement in educational or child development settings. Through these experiences, the longitudinal and social aspects of development and their implications for management become more apparent. In fact, in the training program described by Richardson, Guralnick, and Tupper (1978), most of the residents commented on the unique and important perceptions they were able to obtain from observing and interacting with children and staff in a preschool program.

Existing Collaborative Efforts

Despite the apparent value of increased collaboration between special education and pediatric training, the available data suggest that only limited interactions are occurring. For example, in 1977 a survey of 324 pediatric residency program directors was conducted to determine if opportunities were provided to pediatric residents to observe handicapped children in educational settings. Of the 204 program directors responding, approximately 40% indicated no involvement in educational settings, and only 20% indicated experiences that were formal and required.

In order to obtain another estimate of the relationship between special education and medicine in general, we surveyed most major student-oriented textbooks in special education at various levels from 1970 to the present. The results indicated that very little is said about the collaboration of medical professionals and special educators. As might be expected, most of the instances that were noted centered on specific medical problems of handicapped children.

Finally, in order to determine what professionals in special education are saying to each other regarding relationships with physicians, three major journals related to special education were reviewed. The titles of all articles from 1970 to the present in *The Journal of Special Education, Exceptional Children,* and *The American Journal of Orthopsychiatry* were examined to determine if they were concerned with any aspect of medicine. Those articles that suggested a possibility of being relevant were examined more closely. The results of this analysis revealed that while there is involvement of medical concepts and consultations in the special education process, there is generally little concern with communication between physicians and special educators about the educational process or program planning. That is, the interaction between these two groups that is discussed in the professional literature is typically in regard to specific medical problems that might be experienced by exceptional children or that describes medical input into specific diagnostic processes. There were occasional articles by physicians that were written to benefit educators, but there were no articles specifically concerned with a collaboration (e.g., mutual training efforts) or communication (e.g., involvement in the team process) between physicians and special educators.

CONCLUSIONS

Perhaps the most striking aspect of the material reviewed in this chapter is the high level of agreement in terms of the services that the pediatrician should provide to handicapped children and their families and of the training needs in this area. Given this agreement, the question remains as to how to develop and implement such training programs. Some of the broad strokes with regard to content are outlined in this chapter, as well as some suggested training and evaluation strategies. However, it appears that, above all, a coherent, well-defined, and organized curriculum is essential; it must be flexible and adaptable to the various training levels, it must lend itself to evaluation, and it must be generally accepted if significant progress is to occur. As is seen in the remaining chapters of this book, initial efforts in this direction are underway. However, the next few years will determine whether adequate support, continued interest, and sufficient resources can be mobilized to complete this major and vital undertaking.

REFERENCES

Battle, C. U. 1972. The role of the pediatrician as ombudsman in the health care of the young handicapped child. Pediatrics, 50, 916–921.

Beck, G., Edgar, E., Kenowitz, L., Sulzbacher, W., Lovitt, T., and Zweibel, S. 1978. The physician-educator team: Let's make it work. Journal of School Health, 48, 79–83.

Begab, M. J. 1971. Mental retardation and family stress. In F. J. Menolascino (Ed.), Psychiatric Aspects of Diagnosis and Treatment of Mental Retardation. Seattle: Special Child Publications.

Begab, M. J., and Richardson, S. A. (Eds.). 1975. The Mentally Retarded and Society: A Social Science Perspective. Baltimore: University Park Press.

Bradley, C. 1953. Medical education in mental deficiency. American Journal of Mental Deficiency, 58, 310–315.

Cooke, R. E. 1966. Residency training — A summary of the findings of the PREP Committee. Pediatrics, 38, 720-725.

de la Cruz, F. 1976. Pediatric care and training: A paradox? In T. D. Tjossem (Ed.), Intervention Strategies for High Risk Infants and Young Children. Baltimore: University Park Press.

Farber, B. 1975. Family adaptations to severely mentally retarded children. In M. J. Begab and S. A. Richardson (Eds.), The Mentally Retarded and Society: A Social Science Perspective. Baltimore: University Park Press.

Fishler, K., Koch, R., Sands, R., and Bills, J. 1968. Attitudes of medical students toward mental retardation: A preliminary study. Journal of Medical Education, 43, 64-68.

Gorham, K. A., Des Jardins, C., Page, R., Pettis, E., and Scheiber, B. 1975. Effect on parents. In N. Hobbs (Ed.), Issues in the Classification of Children (Vol. 2). San Francisco: Jossey-Bass.

Helfer, R. E. 1970. An objective comparison of the pediatric interviewing skills of freshman and senior medical students. Pediatrics, 45, 623-627.

Hobbs, N. 1975. The Futures of Children. San Francisco: Jossey-Bass.

Jacobs, H. J., and Walker, D. K. 1978. Pediatricians and The Education for All Handicapped Children Act of 1975 (Public Law 94-142). Pediatrics, 61, 135-137.

Johnston, R. B. 1976. Medicine. In R. B. Johnston and P. R. Magrab (Eds.), Developmental Disorders: Assessment, Treatment, Education. Baltimore: University Park Press.

Johnston, R. B., and Magrab, P. R. 1976. Introduction to developmental disorders and the interdisciplinary process. In R. B. Johnston and P. R. Magrab (Eds.), Developmental Disorders: Assessment, Treatment, Education. Baltimore: University Park Press.

Kelly, N. K., and Menolascino, F. J. 1975. Physicians' awareness and attitudes toward the retarded. Mental Retardation, 13, 9-13.

Koch, R., and Kugel, R. B. (Eds.). 1971. The Pediatrician and the Child with Mental Retardation. Committee on Children with Handicaps. Evanston, Ill.: American Academy of Pediatrics.

Oster, J. 1974. Training of medical and dental students in mental retardation. Acta Paediatrica Scandinavica, Supplement, 246, 1-37.

Palfrey, J. D., Mervis, R. C., and Butler, J. A. 1978. New directions in the evaluation and education of handicapped children. New England Journal of Medicine, 298, 819-824.

Pearson, P. H. 1968. The physician's role in diagnosis and management of the mentally retarded. Pediatric Clinics of North America, 15, 835-859.

Pilkington, T. L. 1977. Teaching medical students about mental handicap. Developmental Medicine and Child Neurology, 19, 652-658.

President's Committee on Mental Retardation. 1977. MR 76 Mental Retardation: Past and Present. Washington D.C.: U.S. Government Printing Office.

Richardson, H. B., and Guralnick, M. J. 1978. Pediatric residents and young handicapped children: Curriculum evaluation. Journal of Medical Education, 53, 487-492.

Richardson, H. B., Guralnick, M. J., and Tupper, D. B. 1978. Training pediatricians for effective involvement with handicapped preschool children and their families. Mental Retardation, 16, 3-7.

Simeonsson, R. J., Kenny, W., and Walker, L. 1976. Child development and disability: Competency-based clerkship. Journal of Medical Education, 51, 578-581.

Solomons, G., and Menolascino, F. J. 1968. Medical counseling of parents of the retarded. Clinical Pediatrics, 7, 11–16.

Tarjan, G. 1976. The Role of Higher Education in Mental Retardation and Other Developmental Disabilities. Report of the Long-Range Task Force on University Affiliated Facilities funded from DHEW under Contract #100-75-0150.

The Task Force on Pediatric Education. 1978. The Future of Pediatric Education. Evanston, Ill.: American Academy of Pediatrics.

chapter 2

PEDIATRIC EDUCATION AND EXCEPTIONAL CHILDREN
A Federal Perspective

Vince L. Hutchins and William W. Swan

Nearly 50 years ago at the 1930 White House Conference on Children, the 13th objective in the Children's Charter stated:

> For every child who is blind, deaf, crippled, or otherwise physically handicapped, and for the child who is mentally handicapped, such measures as will early discover and diagnose his handicap, provide care and treatment, and so train him that he may become an asset to society, rather than a liability (Bremner, 1971, p. 107).

This book (and the conference upon which much of it is based), with its emphasis on curricula for pediatricians on the needs of exceptional children, is another step toward the attainment of that objective. A premise underlying the design of these curricula is that a broadly trained pediatrician must have the ability to identify, to assess, and to treat the exceptional child, and should have the capacity to utilize and interrelate other resources in planning with the family for the child's future.

FEDERAL LEGISLATION AND PROGRAMS

In many respects, the information contained in the chapters of this book parallels the considerable degree of federal activity, from both legislative and program standpoints, that has occurred in the last few years. Of course, the most significant piece of legislation has been the Education for All Handicapped Children Act of 1975 (PL 94-142). This act mandates a free appropriate public education for all handicapped children from 3 to

18 years of age by September, 1978, and for children from 3 to 21 years of age by September, 1980. The law provides detailed statements on the rights of children and their parents, confidentiality, responsibilities of the local and state education agencies, private schools and their participation, procedural safeguards, evaluation of children, placement procedures, program evaluation, and detailed use of funds, to mention but a few.

Perhaps one of the most significant programmatic features of the law is the requirement for the development of an Individualized Education Program (IEP) for each child. The IEP requires parent participation and approval prior to and during its implementation. The content of the IEP includes statements regarding the child's present level of educational performance, annual goals including short-term instructional objectives, the specific special education and related services to be provided to the child, the extent to which the child will be able to participate in regular educational programs, the projected dates for initiation of services, the anticipated duration of the services, the evaluation procedures, the objective evaluation criteria, and the schedules for determining on at least an annual basis whether the short-term instructional objectives are being achieved. Related services may include health services, counseling services, adapted physical education, transportation, recreational activities, special interest groups or clubs sponsored by a public agency, and referrals to other agencies.

PL 94-142 is most emphatic in recognizing the rights of handicapped children and their parents and the responsibilities of the agencies serving these children and their families (Abeson and Zettel, 1977). Furthermore, the law provides for state departments of education to provide an annual plan that responds to each of the criteria specified in the regulations. Consistent with the specificity of the regulations, one division of the Bureau of Education for the Handicapped (Assistance to States) has been assigned to determine if states are complying with the law. The law and the associated regulations significantly focus on the uniqueness of the individual child within the educational system.

Programmatically, the focus on young handicapped children is administered through the Handicapped Children's Early Education Program of the Bureau of Education for the Handicapped (DeWeerd and Cole, 1976). New developments in this program include model efforts that emphasize the infant and the family and cooperative efforts with neonatal intensive care units, cross-age tutoring, utilizing senior citizens as integral parts of treatment teams, serving minority children, enhancing minority leadership, longitudinal investigations of selected aspects of early childhood education for the handicapped, increased efforts in validating particular curriculum models with additional training efforts focusing on approved models, and assisting state education agencies in implementing early childhood state plans.

Physician Involvement

Since comprehensive service cannot occur without effective and knowledgeable physician involvement, a significant component of these new efforts is to contribute to physician training in relation to young handicapped children. Specifically, since it is often the physician who is the first person to see the handicapped child or to be sought out by concerned parents to "help" a potentially handicapped child, the role of the physician is essential in early detection and associated treatment. Furthermore, the pediatrician often provides the first entry point for obtaining appropriate services for a handicapped child and his/her family. With such a responsibility, however, the physician needs to obtain the knowledge of the variety of services and resources that might be available. All of this involvement clearly implies the necessity for extensive training in the developmental and behavioral aspects of pediatrics.

In a review of the Education for All Handicapped Children Act of 1975, Palfrey, Mervis, and Butler (1978) make an important point with regard to physician involvement. They note that this legislation focuses professional attention

> ...on the performance and potential of handicapped children...in effect, mandates physicians to expand their [own] training...fosters better communication between medicine and education... [encourages] multidisciplinary decision-making... and help[s] parents deal [with a new role of participation in their child's evaluation] (pp. 823-824).

Moreover, recent health legislation has emphasized the concepts of accountability and individualization. For example, the Supplemental Security Income Amendments of 1976 mandate the development of individual care plans for the eligible blind and disabled children. These care plans must include appropriate plans for health services, educational services, habilitation services, and social services. The plan, then, must be developed across disciplines and across agencies. Legislation establishing the Hemophilia Treatment Program also requires that individual care plans be developed for these children. These legislative acts detailing individual care plans are unique in health legislation.

IMPLEMENTATION STRATEGIES AND EVALUATION

A strategy in education has been defined as a "means for causing an advocated innovation to become successfully installed in an ongoing educational system" (Miles, 1964). The first steps toward the ultimate implementation of this advocated innovation — the proposed curriculum change in pediatric training that is needed to standardize the teaching of human development and exceptional children — are now occurring through numerous related activities, which include conferences and workshops under a variety of auspices. We expect that these activities will result in complementary guidance that will assist in the next steps of curriculum development and implementation. However, we do recognize that implementation of such a curriculum, even when fully developed, is a complex and difficult process.

For example, a recent article in the nursing literature (Ketefian, 1978) listed several factors that are important for the acceptance and success of a new or modified curriculum. These factors include: commitment of the institution; faculty flexibility; inservice programs for faculty to meet the faculty's learning needs so they can implement the curriculum innovation; participation and involvement of all faculty in the innovation; soundness of the knowledge that constitutes the basis of the innovation; mutual trust among the faculty, between the faculty and their leaders, and between the faculty and the experts that may be used in consultation; and firm leadership that has the authority and acceptance to carry out the implementation.

Consideration must also be given to two other factors. The problem of obtaining time in a medical school for additional curricula is very real and, perhaps, must be part of the institution's commitment. Another factor in the successful implementation of a curriculum on the needs of the exceptional child occurs outside the walls of the training institution. Medical practitioners need to become aware of increasingly complex legislation. Too often in the past there have been gaps in practitioners' knowledge about legislation and the community resources that are available to meet the needs of their patients with complex problems. This information must be included in the practicum aspects of the curricula under discussion.

Thus, with a basis of knowledge of what curricular changes should be made, with firm leadership, and with attention to the factors necessary for success, implementation of the curriculum can be accomplished. Nevertheless, we wish to stress that concurrent with implementation, careful evaluation plans should be developed. The evaluation strategy can be set as the objectives of the program are established. Objectives that are finite and measurable will lend themselves to evaluation more readily than objectives that are general or global. In order for the trainee to achieve the high level of clinical expertise required by the new or modified curriculum, explicit educational objectives are essential for each stage of training. A methodology for setting and evaluating these objectives is presented in the American Board of Pediatrics publication, *Foundations for Evaluating the Competency of Pediatricians* (1974). The chapter by Vaughan (Chapter 6), as well as chapters by others in this volume, describe this potentially useful methodology — the tasks by abilities matrix.

Certainly there is a concern in Congress that handicapped children have not been receiving the comprehensive and integrated services that they require. To be responsive to this congressional challenge and to the needs of our patients, systematic cooperative implementation and evaluation strategies must occur. The curricula that are developed should go beyond training in the traditional areas of clinical expertise of the physician to include the ability to develop and monitor a long-term plan, the ability to work with multidisciplinary teams, the ability to utilize community resources, and finally, the ability to set functional goals and, thus, to influence patient outcome.

REFERENCES

Abeson, A., and Zettel, J. 1977. The end of the quiet revolution: The Education for All Handicapped Children Act of 1975. Exceptional Children, 44, 114–128.

American Board of Pediatrics, Inc. 1974. Foundations for Evaluating the Competency of Pediatricians. Chicago: American Board of Pediatrics, Inc.

Bremner, R. H. (Ed.). 1971. Children and Youth in America: A Documentary History (Vol. 2, Parts 1–6) Cambridge, Mass.: Harvard University Press.

DeWeerd, J., and Cole, A. 1976. Handicapped children's early education program. Exceptional Children, 43, 155–157.

The Education for All Handicapped Children Act of 1975. 1977. P.L. 94-142, Federal Register 42(163): 42474–42518.

Ketefian, S. 1978. Strategies of curriculum change. International Nursing Review, 25, 217.

Miles, M. B. 1964. Innovation in Education. New York: Teachers College Press.

Palfrey, J. S., Mervis, R. C., and Butler, J. A. 1978. New directions in the evaluation and education of handicapped children. New England Journal of Medicine, 298, 819–824.

chapter 3

EDUCATING PHYSICIANS IN CHILD DEVELOPMENT
Why, What, and How

Nicholas J. Anastasiow and Arthur H. Stengel

THE "WHY"

In the early 1960s, dramatic changes began to take place in the field of child growth and development (C-G/D). Many of the then popular "truths" about children and how they grow into adults came under serious attack. The acceptance in the United States of Piaget (1970) and his notion that the child is not a miniature adult, but rather a dynamic being who constantly interacts with, yet remains dependent upon, the environment for intellectual growth, provided the initial force for this shift. Further breakthroughs by American, Scottish, and Russian researchers forever destroyed the notion of the incompetent infant (Stone, Smith, and Murphy, 1973). The infant who had been perceived as born helpless was now perceived as born active, competent, and, in many ways, in control of his/her own learning. Furthermore, and still more recently, evolutionary theorists concluded that the human being is born ready to learn and that the push to learn is the product of a genetic mutation (Jerison, 1976).

The momentum generated by early research and theorizing continues today. Several independent longitudinal studies conducted by physicians and psychologists in the United States and England indicate that whether an infant who lived through perinatal stress functions as a "normal" school-age child is more dependent on social, rather than physiological, factors. Work at the University of Colorado Medical School (Emde, Gaensbauer, and Harmon, 1976) provided new insights and understanding into the issues of regularity and continuity of growth and development. Additional studies and details of these discoveries are discussed in the next section. For now, it is sufficient to note that the revolution in

C-G/D continues today to add new and exciting knowledge for use in the understanding and care of infants and children.

Training Programs for Physicians

If we look into training programs for pediatricians, we find that pediatrics has grown beyond a specialty training that focuses on the treatment of the acute and infectious disorders of children. To a greater and greater extent, the processes of child development are considered the theoretical base upon which many aspects of pediatrics should rest (The Task Force on Pediatric Education, 1978). A recent survey by the American Academy of Pediatrics regarding residency training programs indicated that there are some efforts to include an adequate C-G/D curriculum, but these programs are not as widespread as would be expected given the general acceptance of the relevance of developmental processes to pediatric practice. In fact, more recent graduates of pediatric training are quick to confess, and not without a degree of uneasiness, that they know little of child growth and development save for the infant's physical development and what child growth and development they were able to cram the night before examinations. As Richmond (1975) notes, from a "...perspective of more than twenty years of effort of attempting to teach child development in pediatrics it is unfortunately necessary to record we still have a long way to go" (p. 523).

Medical School Curriculum   The desire to include a C-G/D curriculum has had its peaks and valleys in medical school. A C-G/D curriculum that emphasized Gesellian motor development became part of medical training in the early decades of this century. In our interviews with physicians, we find that many who graduated during this period are conversant with the Gesell books on growth and development. Moreover, in some centers during the 1950s, development was expanded to include psychosocial issues. However, the emphasis remained on physical growth with an occasional lecture on child psychiatry (Gordon, 1976).

It is our contention that one of the reasons why development was deemphasized in medical schools was that the knowledge available from the field of growth and development in 1950 had been integrated into the general culture and was well known and considered common sense. Most medical students had become acquainted with the general principles contained in Spock and in Gesell from their families and/or high school courses. For example, the basic Gesellian notion of ontogenic growth, which stressed physical growth and the genetic push toward completing growth by maturation, was generally accepted as fact by middle class families. Babies were perceived to mature on their own and at roughly similar rates. Charts, readily available in Spock (1957) and Gesell (1954), could be consulted to determine developmental milestones for sitting, crawling, walking, and other global accomplishments. The general opinion of how to facilitate growth was to feed, clothe, clean, bathe, inoculate, and love the infant, in that order. Advice for mothers was readily available from most magazines, many of them found in the physicians' waiting room (Anastasiow, 1978). From our interviews, we conclude that there was no felt need to include such common knowledge in a formal curriculum, and thus the C-G/D curriculum remained focused on motor development.

Two concepts appear to have remained from this early focus. The first is an emphasis on physical growth and development. Increasing stress continues to be placed on the measurement of the presence or absence of reflexes as a sign of normal or abnormal development (St. Clair, 1978), and assessing physical growth and development remains a major diagnostic tool (Touwen, 1976). The Apgar screening device appeared to gain acceptance in the 1950s and has remained a regular part of newborn screening (St. Clair, 1978). Moreover, the appearance of the Denver Developmental Screening Test (Frankenburg and Dodds, 1967) and its distribution to all medical students and physicians throughout the country in 1967, made a major inroad in stressing C-G/D norms. It should be noted, however, that the instrument follows the medical model of "looking for pathology" (Frankenburg, 1978).

Second, it was not uncommon for the medical school curriculum to include an occasional or planned series of lectures from psychiatry, which focused on disorders that arose from severe psychosocial deprivation or grossly abnormal adult-child interactions such as physical and sexual abuse (Goldfarb, 1945). These experiences remained heavily at the abstract level and did not, typically, delve into the clinical realm of social disorders or psychosocial development.

Changing Concepts in Developmental Disorders

As valuable as the knowledge of physical development, reflex measurement, and determining the impact of severe psychosocial deprivation are, they are not sufficient in themselves. That is, additional knowledge is needed to equip the physician to detect the developmental problems that are associated with less severe deficits in the psychosocial environment or to identify and treat disorders, either genetic or stress-related in origin, which display themselves in a subtle fashion in the course of development.

A dramatic example of the change in knowledge and attitudes in C-G/D is the bizarre and still poorly understood disorder of infantile autism. The nature of this disorder allows us to dramatize the point that it is essential to add new techniques to the physician's diagnostic repertoire.

Infantile autism is a serious disorder that typically has not been detected until around the second year of the child's life (Rimland, 1964). The major indicator of the disorder has been the absence of spoken language, which usually becomes fully apparent at that time. In addition to being difficult to detect during infancy, autism has been suggested as being related to parents' inadequacies in relating to children (Kanner, 1949).

Today, it is more commonly assumed that autism is associated with a neurologic disorder of unknown etiology, but the indicators of the disorder are now being detected much earlier. Autistic children appear to have slower responses to spoken patterns of speech than normal children (Condon, 1975), tend to avert rather than hold mother's gaze (Hutt and Ounsted, 1966), and have distinctive crying patterns (Ricks, 1975). All of the above deviations in development present themselves in infancy. More specifically, Ricks (1975) reports that mothers could readily identify at least four meanings in the cries of their normal infants: requests, frustration, greetings, and surprise-pleasure. However, while the mothers could identify the meaning of the cry, they could not identify their own child's cries from the cries of other children or from the cries of children of foreign-speaking parents. With autistic children, the results are startlingly different. Mothers of autistic children could easily identify the distinctive pattern of their autistic child's cries, as well as the meaning of the cries of normal infants. Thus, these mothers may detect an irregularity in their child's crying that is predictive of developmental disorders and that occurs by the time the child is 3 months old. It is not uncommon for these mothers to attempt to communicate their discomfort with their child's development to a physician. Often these mothers have had other normal children and the differences in this infant are clear to them (Brazelton, 1975). The physician must be sensitive to the potential value of the mother's observations.

This newer knowledge of the indicators of autism has shattered many previous notions of infant incompetence, and the physician who possesses the new norms can more readily respond to parents' legitimate concerns. It would appear that there are at least three facets to the problem that result from a failure to incorporate an up-to-date C-G/D curriculum into the training of physicians. First, the vast amount of highly current knowledge about child growth and development will not be made available to them. Second, and stemming from the lack of knowledge, physicians will rely on old "common sense" opinions about children, which in many respects are seriously outmoded and potentially damaging to the child. Third, in addition to the newer knowledge itself, refined techniques of assessment that are used to detect potential irregularities in development are now available. Later in this chapter we discuss research that indicates that physicians' diagnostic power is dramatically increased by the addition of psychosocial measures (Werner, Bierman, and French, 1971).

To be sure that we are not perceived as building a straw man, it must be pointed out that there are some medical schools that have consistently taught child development. Individual physicians have labored long to upgrade the child development knowledge of pediatricians. These efforts, however, have not ameliorated the problem. Most physicians are still unaware of the transactional influence of the caregiver and the home (environment) on the infant's development. In the section that follows, we present what we feel are the critical sets of knowledge to be included in a curriculum, whether it be presented during medical school, residency, preceptorships, or continuing education of physicians.

THE "WHAT"

The keys to revising the C-G/D curriculum for pediatricians and other physicians reside in the new perspectives and knowledge that have emerged from the work during the late 1950s and early 1960s. These perspectives — cognitive psychology and the transactional view of development — can be considered as complementary positions, although they come from somewhat independent lines of research. This section briefly discusses these positions that form the theoretical basis for much of the new findings in child growth and development. Other relevant issues to the field of C-G/D are also raised: continuity and variability of development, and the potential impact of the caregiving environment on the growth and development of the child. Throughout these discussions, language development is used as a case in point. Language development was chosen as the focal point because it lends itself nicely to illustration of both theoretical and clinical issues. It should be noted, however, that all of the major issues discussed in this section are relevant and applicable to all areas of child growth and development.

Cognitive and Transactional Perspectives

The infant of the 1970s is viewed as one who is synergistically interacting with the environment. While genetic factors play a dominant role in development, the environment and the caregiver (usually the parent) transact with the infant in a dynamic way to influence and be influenced by the infant's growth and development. This transactional view owes much to the work of Sameroff and Chandler (1975), and stands in contrast to the rather linear and unidirectional view posited by the earlier students of development (e.g., see Gesell, 1954). The basic course of development delineated by these early researchers is not questioned. What is revised is the view of how that development takes place. The relevant questions for today's researcher are: "How, in what ways, and with what relative effectiveness for what age infant do specific dimensions of the mother-infant interaction operate; which effects persist, at what later ages, and how are effects modified or attenuated by intervening experience?'' (Beckwith, 1976, p. 119). With this view of development, one is forced to continually monitor an ever changing *scene*, for it is neither just the star actor — the child — nor the supporting cast — the mother, father, and others — nor the setting that matter. They all do.

In brief, the cognitive position states that a normal child is born with primitive mechanisms (called schemata) that are used to take in information about the environment. The child is born with a set of schemata to learn from and to act upon the environment in order to gather information about the world and how it operates (Gibson, 1977). At birth the child can discriminate color and can scan and track moving objects (Appleton, Clifton, and Goldberg, 1975). The push to learn is genetically programmed and is a lifelong process, with the major accomplishments occurring by the ninth year (Scarr-Salapatek, 1976). The infant is able to not only act upon the environment, but is able to stimulate persons in the environment to respond to his/her activity. By the third month, the infant is able to express physiological and affective needs through crying, smiling, and vocalizing. In essence, the child is able to communicate with the significant person available in the environment (Lewis and Rosenblum, 1977). Caregivers (usually the mother) appear to be genetically programmed to respond to the infant's communication patterns (Rossi, 1978). Mothers respond to smiles and quickly learn the meaning of infant cries, which vary from hunger and distress to comfort and attention seeking (Wolff, 1969). Infants appear to turn stimulation on and off through sleep and awake states, which vary from awake-alert, awake-active, and awake-quiet to doze, light sleep, or deep sleep (Eisenberg, 1976). They are able to engage the caregiver in eye gaze contact and to hold the gaze of the caregiver (Bower, 1974). Furthermore, the infant is able to make perceptual discriminations, which favor speech sounds over voices or music and happy speech over angry or harsh speech.

Of major importance is the fact that the infant is born learning and that he/she learns very complex facts at early ages. For example, in a very interesting experiment, infants were reinforced by having sets of colored lights go on if they turned their heads in the direction the experimenter wished (Papousek, 1969). They readily learned this act and looked as if they took pleasure in doing so. The experimenter noted that after the lights went on the infant did not particularly watch the lights, but he/she appeared to want to turn them on again. The infant's satisfaction appeared to come from the ability to control the environment by making the lights come on. At times when an infant turned correctly and the lights did not come on, the infant frowned, appeared puzzled, and eventually was cross. It is the need to *learn about, control,* and *predict* how the environment acts that the infant appears to be programmed to learn. Once learning has occurred, expectations of how things operate serve as a fundamental principle of development and appear to operate as a major strategy for infants (and adults as well) (Bandura, 1978).

Thus, the social environment of persons and things transacts with the infant's initial schemata to enable the child to learn through his/her activities. These learnings modify the primitive schemata into more complex ones and, over the course of the next few years, the learnings evolve into more complex mechanisms that guide attention, perception, and thought processes (Piaget, 1971; Neisser, 1967, 1976).

Language Development as a Model

In the case of language development, the ability to smile, to gaze, and to make vocalizations (cooing and babbling) appear to stimulate an adult to talk to the infant (Bloom and Lahey, 1978). Babbling per se is not talking and is not directly related to the later speech of the child (Lenneberg, 1967). Rather, the production of these sounds appears to provide the caregiver with sounds that can be shaped into words of the social environment into which the child has been born, and to engage the adult in interactions. An infant who emits an "i" as in "hi" may be provided with the "hi" by an American mother. The same "i" may be ignored by a British mother. Conversely, the British mother may respond to the "lo" as in "hello" and repeat that word for the infant. Interestingly, the babbling of infants at 3 months contains the same sounds whether the child is born into a Russian, American, Chinese, or any other home. By 6 months, the babbling becomes limited to the sounds of the social environment (Irwin and Chen, 1946). Moreover, these early interactions, both verbal and nonverbal, appear to form the basis of a communicative network upon which later language develops (Bruner, 1975; Freedle and Lewis, 1977).

Some researchers have recently posited the presence of a "feature detector" by which infants can detect sounds (Eimas, 1974). Marler (1977) has proposed an auditory "template" by which the infant can match incoming sounds with the sounds he/she can produce. It is suggested that through this matching process the infant systematically learns to favor those sounds that are present in the environment and to eliminate those that are not. Caregivers seem to respond to what the infant is engaged in and provide words that call attention to the object or activity of the infant (Bates, 1976; Bloom and Lahey, 1978; Moerk, 1977; Nelson, 1973). The infant who babbles or coos at a rolling ball may, for example, learn as his/her first word the word provided for a ball. The word itself may not be ball. It may be "roll" or "pretty" or "see."

In general, parents tend to respond to infants in systematic ways that facilitate language development (Bloom and Lahey, 1978; Brown, 1973). They use short simple language with many redundant words or phrases:

"Nice baby. Pretty baby. Nice baby." Their speech draws attention to what the infant is doing or looking at, for example, "See the doggie. Nice doggie. See the doggie. Big doggie." In this sequence of short, simple sentences, the caregiver repeats, rephrases, prompts, and probes. At other times the caregiver may ask and answer his/her own questions: "Where's the baby? Here's the baby. See the baby? Oh, nice baby." It is up to the infant to figure out what the words mean, and normally developing children appear to have a wide range of strategies for doing so (see McLean and Snyder-McLean, 1978).

In partial summary, caregivers enter into a transactional interchange with the infant in language learning and provide the sample of language that is directed to the child. The child is genetically programmed to discriminate speech sounds as early as the first month of life. By the eighth or ninth month, infants can begin to match their own vocalizations with sounds produced by the caregiver. Underlying language development is the sophistication of the schemata present at birth and the reciprocal nature of early child-caregiver interactions. Let us step back and trace the acquisition of one word and see how the actual spoken word may have been acquired.

Acquisition of the first word   At birth, about 5%–10% of the infant's awake time is spent scanning the environment, and this time increases to 35% by 3 months of age (Bloom and Lahey, 1978). As noted earlier, the infant can discriminate among colors and can follow moving objects. By 2 to 4 months, infants will anticipate the emergence of a moving object from a screen behind which they have seen it move (Bower, 1974). They will anticipate the path of the object to be regular and will follow any object that emerges on the path whether it is the original object or not.

In addition, the infant's selective listening is maturing very rapidly. By 3 months, the child's preference for human speech over music or noise matures further into a preference for mother's voice. At 4 months, infants are able to detect mother's footsteps (Eisenberg, 1976). By 3 months, the infant has mastered the art of smiling and is now able to control smiling and to smile at mother and persons and things that give him/her pleasure (Emde et al., 1976). Communication occurs through crying, thrashing, vocalizing, gazing, and smiling.

Caregivers, in turn, provide toys that attract infants. In an interesting experiment, Rovee and Rovee (1969) demonstrated that not only are infants able to control a mobile that is attached to their leg by a string, but they will learn to kick faster if the mobile moves faster in response to the kicking rate. Infants can learn how to do this as early as 2 to 4 months of age.

Development is a combination and integration of the simple behaviors, present at birth, into complex behaviors (Appleton, Clifton, and

Goldberg, 1975). As Werner and Kaplan (1963) postulate, development moves from simple to complex, with finer and finer discriminations made leading to categorization and hierarchical organization of knowledge. All of the skills that the infant has are used first to find out what a thing is and does and *then* to learn the name for it. At 7 to 9 months, the infant is able to respond fully to the meaning of verbal messages, such as, "Show me a big smile" (Zelazo, 1972). Also by this time, an elaborate communications network has been established through caregiver-child interactions. Even prelinguistically, through reciprocal social interactions, the groundwork for language use (pragmatics) and aspects of its grammar have emerged (Bruner, 1975). It is at this time that the first word usually appears.

The caregiver in our earlier example has provided the infant with a ball. The ball is rolled and bounced while the caregiver says: "See the ball. Pretty ball. Nice ball." After having these experiences, and at around 9 to 12 months of age, the infant may emit his first word, "ball." The child may then call all things that roll "ball," such as toy cars. Nelson (1973) found, for example, that children whose caregivers labeled snacks as "cookies" had children who learned to call "cookie" all foods they liked for snacks, such as fruit and celery, and they labeled all foods they did not like as "no cookie" (which might in some cases include actual cookies). These first words fall into two general categories. The first category is the names of objects and people. The second category is function words, such as "go," when the child wants to go out or have something, or "gone," when the child has finished dinner.

From 12 months to the second year, children's speech is dominated by things and events. By 24 months, two-word sentences appear, and by 36 months more complex sentences appear reflecting more complex reasoning and inference making. Throughout, language development is the product of a complex set of interactions that have a cognitive and social base. Language development continues in a regular sequence with the major accomplishment of mastering the basic syntax, the morphology, and the phonology of one's native language completed by the age of 5 or 6 (McNeill, 1970). This acquisition appears to be universally accomplished at the same age period by all children across all cultures, with the exception of some difficult to pronounce forms (such as the double consonant in medial positions as in "twelfth") that are not mastered until about 10 years of age (Palermo and Molfese, 1972).

Variability and Continuity in Cognitive Development

A developmental screening instrument is designed to sample various behavior areas to detect a potential lag in development. It is designed to suggest whether or not further testing is necessary. The Bayley Scales of Infant Development (1969) or the Brazelton Neonatal Behavioral Assessment Scale (1973) are examples of such follow-up diagnostic instruments. Each instrument is built on the assumption of the similarity of growth patterns and rates across infants. Given an adequate environment and a facilitating caregiver (both are described in the section that follows), normal infants resemble each other more than they differ. However, two factors must be kept in mind. First, infants vary in the pace of development and they vary from day to day in how they perform. Eisenberg's (1976) work suggests that the "awake-alert" state may be the most ideal and accurate period for measuring the infant's competencies.

The second source of variability exists among the different competencies that the infant possesses. Competencies mature at varying rates — visual discrimination may preceed the maturation of the auditory feature detector. However, the normal infant's global score on a test reflects these variable growth rates, which the individual assessments by a physician must take into account. In general, the delayed youngster will be uniformly lower on all functions, and the normal child shows relatively minor peaks and valleys. This is why so many abilities are attained across a span of months.

The first year of life is very old genetically and is rigidly programmed biologically (Scarr-Salapatek, 1976). The intensity of the biological program is such that it takes a major environmental or intrauterine disruption to change the regular flow of events. Thus, babies mature at similar rates and acquire similar sets of skills and abilities at about the same time. However, within this regular progression, some fundamental biobehavioral shifts do occur. In a longitudinal study of infants, Emde et al. (1976) found two such shifts occurring in the first year of life. The first shift occurs at 2 to 3 months and is best characterized by the development of the social smile from a smile that appears with REM (rapid eye movement) sleep and awake states. The smiling capacity becomes generalized to all objects at 1½ to 2 months, and by 3 to 3½ months the infant appears to be able to control the smile. This capacity is accompanied by increasing wakeful states, decreased fussiness, and decreased awake REM states. There are marked differences in electroencephalographic patterns as well.

The next major shift is at 7 to 9 months when the infant demonstrates a fear of strangers. The fear signals the infant's ability to discriminate a stranger from a non-stranger. As in the earlier shift, increasing periods of wakefulness preceed the biobehavioral change. Other shifts probably occur in early childhood, but far less is known about them.

The most dramatic school-age shift about which a great deal is known is the one that occurs between 5 to 7 years of age. White (1965) has catalogued sets of discrete abilities that the 7-year-old possesses that were not present just prior to the shift.

At the biological level Epstein (1974) has suggested that increased myelinization of the brain may occur at periods correlated with rapid developmental growth. In a study of three sets of autopsy data, Epstein (1974, 1978) found a correspondence in the growth spurts of the brain across the three samples. These spurts occur at 3 to 10 months, 2 to 4 years, 6 to 8 years, 10 to 12 years, and 14 to 16 years. He notes that these growth spurts closely match norms of mental tests for the general population. Epstein speculates that the periods of training and intervention might best occur during these periods when the brain axons and dendrites are increasing in length and branching. It is interesting to note that the final sheathing of the corpus callosum by age 10 matches Epstein's next to last stage, and that the final growth of the brain is usually complete by age 15, Epstein's last stage (Rudel, 1978).

Epstein's stages of brain growth parallel in some ways the age-stage theory of cognitive development by Piaget (1970). Piaget's stages include the sensorimotor period, 0–2 years; preoperational thought, 2–7 years (preoperational phase, 2–4 years; intuitive phase, 4–7 years); concrete operations, 7–11 years; and formal operations, 11–15 years. Although a rough similarity exists between the biopsychological theory of Piaget and Epstein's data, the key point is that the stage concept of development is supported at many levels of analysis.

Biobehavioral reorganizations may be one reason why the so-called infant IQ measures fail to predict later IQ scores (Honzig, 1976). That is, infants make the shift over a 1- or 2-month period, and functioning previous to the shift is of a different qualitative nature than the functioning that follows. The test administered prior to the shift will result in markedly different results.

A second hypothesis of why infant IQ measures do not predict later IQ is tied to the basic genetic nature of development in the first 2 years. Intelligence tests during school years measure social knowledge — vocabulary, solving problems, analogies, and so on. However, the first 18 months (the sensorimotor period) have a strong genetic-biological base that is resistant to all but the most extreme social influences (Scarr-Salapatek, 1975). Nevertheless, even though all normal infants tend to complete the sensorimotor period in pretty much the same way, changes in learning strategies, social prerequisites for learning, and other developmental patterns can be significantly affected by social influences.

A third reason that infant IQ measures are not good predictors is that they are single status measures of the infant (cognitive) and that they fail to assess the environment and the skills of the major agent in the environment, usually the mother. Uniformly, studies that have chosen one variable as a "main effect" to predict infant attainments have failed. Infant development is genetically programmed but is dependent upon an environment and an agent in the environment. As we discuss below, the agent can facilitate development by the manner in which he/she transacts with the child. In this sense we have called the mother-caregiver/agent a facilitator.

The Facilitator

The transactional nature of caregiver-infant behavior has been emphasized throughout this chapter. In this section, the facilitating nature of the transactional relationships is focused upon. We have seen that the infant can express his/her feelings early in life and finds pleasure in controlling the environment. In many ways the infant is an affective behavior system (Scarr-Salapatek, 1975).

The importance of a consistent person who serves as caregiver was well documented by Spitz (1945, 1946) and Bowlby (1969). Children who have prolonged separation from the caregiver suffered developmental delays, which in many cases were very difficult to remediate (Clarke and Clarke, 1977). The value of a consistent caregiver is complex given the intricate series of interrelations established between the mother and the child, perhaps beginning even at the earliest point in life. For example, Condon and Sander (1974) have observed that the infant responds to the rhythm of spoken speech almost immediately after birth, and Papousek (1969) has noted that at 7 days of age, although the infant cannot recognize all the features of mother's face, he/she expresses a startle (or surprise) response if mother wears a surgical mask.

The infant and primary caregiver become "attached" or "bonded" in the early days of the infant's life, and it appears that bonding facilitates development (Bowlby, 1969; Brazelton, 1969). Just how this occurs is a matter of speculation at this writing. However, a great deal is known about those child-rearing attitudes that facilitate development. In a summary of more than 60 separate studies, Martin (1975) reports a consistent pattern of attitudes on the part of those parents whose children succeed in school, i.e., those children who have higher IQ scores and higher achievement tests scores. The "successful" techniques are a moderate use of warmth, a high level of verbalization or talking to the child, a high use of reasoning, a low use of physical punishment, and a press for developmental attainments. These parents provide an environment that responds to their children's needs but presses the children to make age appropriate attainments.

Further support for this can be found in the works of Heiniche (1976) and Baumrind (1972). They noted that development is facilitated by parents who provide for independence and exploration in an atmosphere of support and who have the expectation that the child will master age appropriate tasks. Heiniche refers to the accomplishment as *task orientation*. As we have seen, children may be motivated to learn through evolutionary pressures. Parental action facilitates the achievement of specific environmental tasks that are important for the specific culture (eating from a spoon, drinking from a cup) at the time when the child is maturationally ready to master the task. A mismatch of task and maturation is of little consequence if social (parental) pressures are very low and flexibility is high. However, the gross mismatch of task and maturation can be disastrous for the child, as we have come to know from the negative results of harsh and punitive toilet training before 2 years of age.

Let us briefly examine one current study that bears directly on the potential facilitating effects of caregivers. Elardo, Bradley, and Caldwell (1975, 1977) conducted a longitudinal study that measured the child's home environment, as well as developmental, language, and cognitive variables. Their results indicated that scores reflecting the quality of the infant's home environment predicted later IQ twice as accurately as the infant developmental measure. Furthermore, measures of mother's emotional responsiveness and involvement with her infant at 6 months were highly predictive of the child's language development at age 3. However, the mother's demands and responsiveness to the baby change as the baby matures. Thus, these researchers found that the provision of play materials became a critical predictor once the child was a year old. It is surmised that encouragement of independence and exploration arises after the eighth month when the child apparently makes a major biobehavioral shift. Moreover, child-rearing attitudes and associated behavior patterns that lead to school success also appear to be potent remediators of perinatal stress.

Perinatal Stress

It has been well known for at least a hundred years that prematurity and asphyxia following birth are events that may lead to damage of the central nervous system. What was not known was what exactly happened to trigger the central nervous system damage of the premature child and therefore "caused" the associated mental retardation, cerebral palsy, or other handicapping conditions. In the main, speculations as to the causes of the damage focused on the physiological state of the child, yet, Little (in Neligan, Prudham, and Steiner, 1974) anticipated the results found in some of today's studies. Neligan, Prudham, and Steiner quote Little as saying that

> . . . in some instances the weakness of intellect has appeared to result less from permanent injury to the brain than from the want of sufficient training and education after its recovery from the severe physiological shock it had received (p. 1).

Several longitudinal studies were designed to uncover the mechanisms of damage that occurred during the perinatal period, particularly the causes of those conceptual and perceptual deficits found so frequently in school-age children who had suffered perinatal stress (Teuber and Rudel, 1962). We have selected three of the longitudinal studies to be discussed briefly in this chapter: Werner, Bierman, and French's (1971) Kauai study; Neligan, Prudham, and Steiner's (1974) Newcastle upon Tyne study; and Broman, Nichols, and Kennedy's (1975) report on the United States mainland study.

Werner, Bierman, and French, (1971) utilizing tools from pediatrics, psychology, and allied disciplines, observed and documented the course of all the pregnancies and their outcomes in an entire community from the women's first reported menses until her children were 10 years old. The study was designed to assess the effects of perinatal stress on physical, cognitive, and social development of preschool- and school-age children and to evaluate the relative contributions of perinatal stress and the quality of the environment (e.g., maternal well-being, intellectual stimulation, emotional support) to the development of the child (Werner, Bierman, and French, 1971, p. 2). This study complemented and extended previous longitudinal studies in three major respects: all of the children in a multiracial, multiethnic setting were observed; both perinatal stress and quality of the environment were assessed; and observations were begun as early as the fourth week of gestation. The results of the Kauai study were impressive: "Ten times more children had problems attributed to the effects of a poor environment than to the effects of serious perinatal stress" (p. 134). Parental language style, attitudes toward achievement, and involvement and concern had a significant impact on the child before the child reached his/her second birthday. The overwhelming number of children who had suffered severe perinatal stress, but were raised in homes rated favorably in educational stimulation and emotional support, were functioning adequately in school at age 10. In contrast, all children, with one exception, who had suffered severe perinatal stress and were raised in less favorable homes, had serious achievement problems. Thus, parental press for achievement, rich use of language, emotional involvement, and concern for the child appear to dramatically influence and facilitate the child's development before the age of 2.

Neligan, Prudham, and Steiner (1974) reported that the Newcastle upon Tyne study included 13,000 children followed from birth to the age of 10 years. The study differed from the Kauai study in that their measures tended to be more physiologically oriented and their social variables were of a global nature. However, the findings of the Newcastle upon Tyne study were dramatic. The authors state that "the most lethal of perinatal adverse factors which can be directly modified by clinical action (breech delivery and prolonged delay in establishing regular respiration) produce very trivial effects in terms of clinically recognizable signs of brain damage'' (p. 119). Of great significance, the single most important factor in predicting children's IQ was the quality of mother's care as measured during a home visit by a nurse.

The third study is an early report of the well-known collaborative study by Broman, Nichols, and Kennedy (1975). This study included 50,000 women who were identified and followed in 12 medical centers located throughout the United States. The study assessed conditions of pregnancy including physiological, environmental, biological, and genetic factors. The report is detailed and is highly recommended for its elegant treatment of masses of data. The major finding of the study was that the number of years of mother's education and the parents' social class explained most of the variance predictive of the child's IQ at age 4. In her excellent review of the study, Stein (1975) states:

> One is led to ask whether a great deal more will be learned about determinants of IQ in population from further studies in details of pregnancy and birth. To explain environmental related variance in IQ we might better turn our attention towards the postnatal period and the socialization of parents and children (pp. 548–549).

The question can be asked: If parental child-rearing techniques can facilitate, can the converse set of techniques delay development? We believe that they can. The study carried out by Wulbert et al. (1975), comparing language normal children and language delayed children, provides support for this notion. The language delayed children were found to have mothers who were more harsh in their treatment of the child and who tended to use more physical punishment. Furthermore, these mothers frequently ignored their children's requests and seldom praised or caressed their children. In contrast, the language normal children had mothers who were, in addition to the qualities reported above, more verbally and socially interactive with their children.

Implications for Physicians

Werner and Smith (1977), in a follow-up study of the original Kauai children, now age 20, had some very interesting remarks to make to physicians. They noted that when the evaluation for risk status was made by the pediatrician alone, of those children with problems at age 10, only one-half were identified as at-risk as infants. However, when the pediatrician and the psychologist both evaluated the infant, two-thirds of the children who had problems at age 10 were identified. Adding an assessment of the psychosocial variables influencing the child increases the predictive power of an infant assessment. Moreover, Werner's work suggests the use of the following set of predictors for identification in infancy of those children who will not function well at age 10. The first set is the biological state of the infant and includes low birth weight (below 2,000 grams), moderate to severe stress scores, and the presence of a congenital defect at birth. The second set, activity level (or temperament) of the infant, includes low social responsiveness, very high and very low activity, and below 80 Cattell IQ scores. The third set is the social environment, which includes low social economic status, family instability in the first 2 years, and little education of the mother (eighth grade or less).

Finally, given that nonfacilitating parenting skills hinder development, the question can be asked: "Will intervention by a physician help?" The answer is decidedly "Yes." In a carefully controlled study conducted at the University of Colorado, Gray et al. (1977) observed that "abnormal childrearing factors" (what we have referred to as nonfacilitative, i.e., high use of physical punishment, etc.) are correlated with a high incidence of child abuse. Through the use of interview techniques, a questionnaire, and observations of the mother during labor, delivery, and the postpartum period, they were able to identify "high risk mothers for abnormal parenting practices" (p. 1). Half of the high risk group received intervention consisting of comprehensive pediatric services provided by a single pediatrician and a health visitor to the home. The other half of the high risk families received no intervention. The results were impressive. Five cases of child abuse required hospitalization in the nonintervention group, whereas no instances of serious child abuse were found in the intervention group. The observation scales used by Gray et al. (1977) should be of great use to physicians. The point to be made here is that indicators of potential nonfacilitative practices can be observed. These indicators are predictive of abnormal parenting practices that are associated with developmental delays and in some cases child abuse. A pediatrician or other physician, with the aid of a home visitor, can take the first steps to help these mothers develop effective parenting skills and modify their nonfacilitative practices. It is a basic premise of this chapter that the physician's diagnostic power can be increased greatly by adding the skills of detecting and modifying "abnormal" or nonfacilitative child-rearing practices.

In summary, the three studies indicate that the parents influence the child's development during the early months of life in a facilitating or debilitating manner. The impact of the child's early environment is so strong that not only does the mother's manner of child care influence normal development, but it can also reduce the negative effects of perinatal stress. The knowledge of the transactional nature of development and the means to assess the psychosocial environment are essential for pediatricians to possess.

THE "HOW"

The Setting and Instructional Format

"How" knowledge is mastered is closely related to the conditions or setting for learning and the instructional format. Thus, some knowledge is best communicated through one format while other information may be obtained through another. Gagne has done much to specify these "conditions" and we refer to his work in our discussion. We strongly urge the inexperienced trainer to refer to *Conditions of Learning,* 3rd edition, Gagne (1977), and to Gagne and Briggs' *Principles of Instructional Design* (1974) for excellent discussions of the procedures of curriculum development. What follows are some general guidelines of how (and where) knowledge of child growth and development might be developed. We have attempted to analyze situations with which we have become familiar, but we would urge a note of caution. We have discovered unique possibilities in every setting we have visited and suspect there are many other possibilities of which we are unaware. Each curriculum developer must conduct an analysis of his/her own setting to identify the manner, place, and time in which the C-G/D curriculum can be inserted. There are strong biases in every training institution regarding what can or cannot be done. These attitudes, like all human attitudes, are very difficult to change, and we suggest that the trainer select aspects of a C-G/D curriculum that can be inserted into (rather than replace) an ongoing training program in a given setting.

We have observed that the C-G/D curriculum can be inserted during the following periods and activities: medical school class lecture, daily ward rounds, Grand Rounds, attending on ward, attending in nursery and clinic, topical seminar, preceptorships, and fellowships. Interestingly, we began our list with the most restrictive activity (medical school class time where there appears to be little room in the curriculum), and we ended the list with the most flexible activity that can be independently set. A fellowship can be designed to accomplish a wide range of goals similar to what has been discussed here. Brazelton's (1975) program in child development is one such example. (See also Chapter 4, this volume.)

The modes of instruction may vary from lecture, discussion, reading, tutorial, or laboratory practicum (i.e., clinic, ward, office). The materials may vary from books, audiotapes, videotapes, films, and articles, to observations and direct contact. There is a close interaction between these formats and setting conditions and the type of knowledge to be gained.

To clarify this point, let us first assume that the goal is to provide pediatric residents with a general overview of child growth and development. This is aimed at a fairly broad target with an overall "feeling," as opposed to a specific set of skills, as the outcome. Here, one or more readings (e.g., Newman and Newman, 1979) could easily suffice. These readings could be assigned to the resident for discussion at a Grand Rounds or during daily ward rounds.

Now consider this more complex assignment. Assume that the desired goal is to train residents to administer and interpret the Denver Developmental screening instrument. This assignment includes several levels of functioning and requires an involved set of activities. The first level must include assigning the manual to be read, as well as sections from Kazuk, Cohrs, and Frankenburg (1974), which can be completed by residents on their own time and at their own pace. A further extension of training would be to have the resident view the training film on the Denver Developmental Screening Test (LADOCA, 1976) or to observe and discuss an administration by an experienced individual. After this part of the training a set of practice-run administrations of the instrument would further extend the training. Some of this practice can occur, initially, without observation, but later trials should come under careful scrutiny, both regarding administration and interpretation. Since the runs are practice runs, the time for them can be flexibly scheduled. Finally, the resident should administer, score, and interpret several tests in a formal manner while being observed by a skilled practitioner. A nursery or children and youth clinic are good examples of existing settings that can be utilized for this type of training. Furthermore, to maximize the residents' acquisition of a developmental point of view, we suggest that they be assigned to administer the screening device to five children: neonate, 3 months old, 9 months old, 18 months old, and 36 months old. All children should be of the same race and socioeconomic status. These ages are chosen because they are good developmental milestones. This type of training with reading, viewing/listening, and practice with feedback maximizes later performance.

One caveat: the examples just provided do indeed demonstrate how C-G/D can be emphasized within existing settings. It remains critical, however, that one realize that any curriculum change requires careful planning, adequately supported implementation, and competent supervision.

Content and Competencies

Earlier in this chapter we stated that the overall goals of the chapter were to emphasize that the acquisition of new knowledge and refined techniques would greatly increase the physician's diagnostic skills. Furthermore, in the process of obtaining this knowledge, we believe the physician will develop the additional competencies as discussed in this section. The specific curriculum content in child growth and development must blend the theoretical with the practical and the abstract with the concrete. Curriculum development in this area is only at a preliminary level, although the discussion that follows is drawn from our own efforts to develop such a course of study (Anastasiow and Stengel, 1977).

A major goal is to highlight the transactional nature of development played out in an age-stage format. The competencies we have identified stress the ability of the primary care physician to assess the adequacy of an environment composed of the growing child from social, psychological, and physical perspectives. To explain the portion of developmental variance attributed to the environment, attention must be focused on the socialization practices of parents (Stein, 1975). Accordingly, the following educational competencies can be suggested to be part of a curriculum in child development.

Physicians will have a general knowledge of psychosocial development   This knowledge is critical and provides a base from which the physician can make diagnoses and provide suggested plans of treatment or referrals. The physician cannot be expected to become a skilled facilitator of growth unless he/she is aware of the new knowledge in the child development literature. One minor but devastating example may suffice. The physician, unaware of the impact of perceptual and motor activity on brain development (Chall and Mirsky, 1978), may fail to question a parent as to how much time the infant is left unattended in isolated play, a frequent practice of the potentially abusing mother (Gray et al., 1977). This bit of knowledge provides the base from which the physician can generate hypotheses about an infant's apathetic behavior or his/her delayed development. The physician who is aware of the impact of parenting practices in infant development will take time to obtain information from an ecological perspective.

Physicians will have an understanding of the role of screening in the primary care of a child   Screening should accompany regular diagnostic checkups and should include an assessment of the social environment. As we have stressed earlier, how a caregiver interacts with the infant can do much to offset perinatal stress and alter the course of development (Elardo, Bradley, and Caldwell, 1975, 1977; Werner and Smith, 1977). The physician must be sensitive to the precursors of later development, such as the reflexive conversation, which appears to evoke and precede language development.

Screening may be conducted by a paraprofessional or office nurse. Ueda (1978) demonstrated that mothers can fill out a screening form quite adequately and can detect potential problems once given guidance in the form of questions. Although screening has potential problems, the impact of the failure to identify certain disorders early has profound effects on later development. Finally, in expanding the physician's awareness through screening, the physician can become more sensitive to the techniques and methods employed by other professionals in health care and allied fields.

Physicians will have a basic understanding of how to administer and interpret a developmental examination that includes psychosocial issues A physician who has had experience in developmental diagnosis during residency with respect to a range of children from different ethnocultures can appreciate the impact of social class and ethnic child-rearing preferences on children's development. The child-rearing practices that are related to language development, IQ, and school success are generally well known (Martin, 1975). Not all caregivers agree with these strategies (Werner, Bierman, and French, 1971) and the physician who is aware of the impact that these practices have on later development should make an effort to assess them early. In fact, the assessment of the caregiver's knowledge of child-rearing before the infant's birth may do much to reduce developmental delays (Anastasiow et al., 1978).

A physician will possess the basic skills in interviewing adults Throughout this chapter the role of the caregiver in facilitating development has been stressed. The physician must be able to detect those caregivers who, for a variety of reasons, fail to enhance their children's development. An anecdote taken from the authors' observations may be helpful. A very emaciated anemic 14-month-old child was brought to a clinic for a third follow-up examination. The resident expressed alarm and indicated his concern that the latest prescription also seemed not to be ameliorating the problem. He asked the mother about the child's eating habits and the medication. She responded by saying that she administered the medicine and that the child had eaten "some eggs, toast, orange juice, some milk, and a piece of apple." The resident expressed extreme puzzlement. The attending physician asked the mother on what day the child had the orange juice. The mother responded by saying she thought it was last week. Further questioning revealed that the mother concealed her neglectful practices and that the child was fed mainly his bottle and probably had not been administered the medicine. The mother and child were immediately referred to a social worker, who, in that setting, could assume the necessary role of attempting to change the mother's caregiving practices.

For physicians to obtain the competency of detecting the nature of the child-rearing practice, they need to come into contact with allied health care professionals, learn what it is they do, and learn how to utilize their skills. In every setting we observed, there were other support personnel whose expertise was of great potential training value. Social workers are very experienced in moderating the impact of low socioeconomic status on the child's development. A Grand Rounds type lecture by a skilled social worker can do much to explicate the impact of poverty on the child's social, physical, and cognitive development. Similarly, a psychologist who works with the schools possesses invaluable information as to what impact the press of the school has on the child. There are strong psychosocial constraints imposed by the schools, and the failure to live within these constraints, in many cases, leads to the child being referred to special service personnel and often to the pediatrician (Lortie, 1975).

Further Considerations for Content

In some manner the pediatrician should become knowledgeable in the major areas of developmental delay and disability. How to accomplish this is discussed in other chapters of this book. However, we stress the importance of pediatricians coming to recognize that impairments are physical, but that handicaps are social, in nature. That is, handicaps appear when the environment makes demands upon the individual whose impairment does not allow him/her to meet the demands (Carlson, 1976; Mercer, 1973).

Finally, the development of a curriculum should attend to the personal-social development of the pediatrician. Development is life long, and the Life Span Approach is an emerging concept (Vaillant, 1977). One general belief held in psychology is that understanding the child requires adults to be able to put themselves in the place of the child (Loevinger, 1976). The ability to do so requires a moderate degree of self-understanding of one's own stage of psycho-personal growth (Erikson, 1968).

CONCLUSIONS

The role of physicians as primary care providers to families has placed additional demands upon their competencies. Assuming such a role requires that physicians become sophisticated in their ability to assess the dynamic system in which the child and the family reside. This role requires physicians to become aware that not only does the body influence the mind, and the mind the body, but that the social-emotional atmosphere of the environment influences both.

A single chapter such as this must neglect other issues that play a part in the dynamic system, for example, temperamental differences among children, social class as an intervening variable, and race and ethnic differences in child-rearing. It has been our intention to stimulate thought and discussion and to suggest a limited set of knowledge and information in order to provoke interest in detecting psychosocial variables that influence development. We firmly believe that the numbers of handicapped children can be reduced substantially by the thoughtful intervention of the physician early in the child's life.

ACKNOWLEDGMENTS

William K. Frankenburg, M.D., of the University of Colorado Medical School, and William Lupatkin, M.D., of the Columbia-Presbyterian Medical Center, read and commented on a draft of this chapter. We wish to thank them for their comments and suggestions.

REFERENCES

Anastasiow, N. J. 1978. Strategies and models for early childhood intervention programs in integrated settings. In M. Guralnick (Ed.), Early Intervention and the Integration of Handicapped and Nonhandicapped Children. Baltimore: University Park Press.
Anastasiow, N. J., Everett, M., O'Shaughnessy, T. E., Eggleston, P. J., and Eklund, S. J. 1978. Using a child development curriculum to change young teenagers' attitudes toward children, handicapping conditions, and hospital settings. American Journal of Orthopsychiatry, 48(4), 663–672.
Anastasiow, N. J., and Stengel, A. H. 1977. A Mini-Course in Child Development for Pediatricians. Bloomington: Institute for Child Study, Indiana University.
Appleton, T., Clifton, R., and Goldberg, S. 1975. The development of behavioral competence in infancy. In F. D. Horowitz (Ed.), Review of Child Development Research. Chicago: University of Chicago Press.
Bandura, A. 1978. The self system in reciprocal determinism. American Psychologist, 33, 344–358.
Bates, E. 1976. Language and Context: The Acquisition of Pragmatics. New York: Academic Press.
Baumrind, D. 1972. Socialization and instrumental competence in young children. In W. W. Hartup (Ed.), The Young Child: Reviews of Research (Vol. 2). Washington, D.C.: National Association for the Education of Young Children.
Bayley, N. 1969. Bayley Scales of Infant Development. New York: Psychological Corporation.
Beckwith, L. 1976. Caregiver-infant interaction and the development of the high risk infant. In T. Tjossem (Ed.), Intervention Strategies for High Risk Infants and Young Children. Baltimore: University Park Press.
Bloom, L., and Lahey, M. 1978. Language Development and Language Disorders. New York: John Wiley & Sons, Inc.
Bower, T. G. R. 1974. Development in Infancy. San Francisco. W. H. Freeman & Co.
Bowlby, J. 1969. Attachment and loss Vol. 1: Attachment. New York: Basic Books, Inc.
Brazelton, T. B. 1969. Infants and Mothers: Differences in Development. New York: Delacorte Press/Seymour Lawrence.
Brazelton, T. B. 1973. Neonatal Behavioral Assessment Scale. Philadelphia: J. B. Lippincott Co.
Brazelton, T. B. 1975. Training program for pediatricians in child development at the Harvard Medical School. Paper presented at Society for Research in Child Development Meeting, April 17–19, Denver.
Broman, S. H., Nichols, P. L., and Kennedy, W. A. 1975. Preschool IQ. Hillsdale, N.J.: Lawrence Erlbaum Associates.
Brown, R. 1973. A First Language: The Early Stages. Cambridge, Mass.: Harvard University Press.

Bruner, J. S. 1975. The ontogenesis of speech acts. Journal of Child Language, 2, 1-19.

Carlson, N. A. 1976. The Contents of Life: A Socio-Ecological Model of Adaptive Behavior and Functioning. United States Department of Health, Education, and Welfare. Bureau of Education for the Handicapped. East Lansing: Michigan State University.

Chall, J. S., and Mirsky, A. F. (Eds). 1978. Education and the Brain. Chicago: University of Chicago Press.

Clarke, A. D. B., and Clarke, A. M. 1977. Prospects for prevention and amelioration of mental retardation: A guest editorial. American Journal of Mental Deficiency, 81, 523-533.

Condon, W. S. 1975. Multiple response to sound in dysfunctional children. Journal of Autism and Childhood Schizophrenia, 5, 37-56.

Condon, W. S., and Sander, L. W. 1974. Synchrony demonstrated between movements of the neonate and adult speech. Child Development, 45, 456-462.

Eimas, P. D. 1974. Linguistic processing of speech by young infants. In R. L. Schiefelbusch and L. L. Lloyd (Eds.), Language Perspectives — Acquisition, Retardation, and Intervention. Baltimore: University Park Press.

Eisenberg, R. B. 1976. Auditory Competence in Early Life. Baltimore: University Park Press.

Elardo, R., Bradley, R., and Caldwell, B. N. 1975. The relation of infant's home environments to mental tests performance from six to thirty-six months: A longitudinal analysis. Child Development, 46, 71-76.

Elardo, R., Bradley, R., and Caldwell, B. N. 1977. A longitudinal study of the relation of infant's home environment to language development at age three. Child Development, 48, 595-603.

Emde, R. N., Gaensbauer, T. J., and Harmon, R. J. 1976. Emotional Expression in Infancy: A Biobehavioral Study. New York: International Universities Press, Inc.

Epstein, H. T. 1974. Phrenoblysis: Special brain and mind growth periods, Part I: Human brain and skull development; Part II: Human mental development. Developmental Psychobiology, 7, 207-224.

Epstein, H. T. 1978. Growth spurts during brain development: Implication for educational policy and practice. In J. S. Chall and A. F. Mirsky (Eds.), Education and the Brain. Chicago: University of Chicago Press.

Erikson, E. H. 1968. Identity, Youth and Crisis. New York: W. W. Norton & Co., Inc.

Frankenburg, W. K. 1978. Personal communication.

Frankenburg, W. K., and Dodds, J. B. 1967. The Denver developmental screening test. Journal of Pediatrics, 71, 181-191.

Freedle, R., and Lewis, M. 1977. Prelinguistic conversations. In M. Lewis and L. A. Rosenblum (Eds.), Interaction, Conversation, and the Development of Language. New York: John Wiley & Sons, Inc.

Gagne, R. M. 1977. The conditions of learning (3rd ed.). New York: Holt, Rinehart & Winston, Inc.

Gagne, R. M., and Briggs, L. J. 1974. Principles of Instructional Design. New York: Holt, Rinehart & Winston, Inc.

Gesell, A. 1954. The ontogeneses of infant behavior. In L. Carmichael (Ed.), Manual of Child Psychology (2nd Ed.). New York: John Wiley & Sons, Inc.

Gibson, E. J. 1977. How perception really develops: A view from outside the network. In D. LaBerge and S. J. Samuels (Eds.), Basic Processes in Reading: Perception and Comprehension. Hillsdale, N.J.: Lawrence Erlbaum Associates.

Goldfarb, W. 1945. Psychological privation in infancy and subsequent adjustment. American Journal of Orthopsychiatry, 15, 247–255.

Gordon, I. 1976. Personal communication.

Gray, J. D., Cutler, C. A., Dean, J. G., and Kempe, C. H. 1977. Prediction and prevention of child abuse and neglect. Child Abuse and Neglect International Journal, 1, 1–14.

Heiniche, C. M. 1976. Early childhood social and emotional development: Relationship and task orientation. In H. H. Spicker, N. J. Anastasiow, and W. L. Hodges (Eds.), Children with Special Needs: Early Development and Education. Minneapolis: University of Minnesota.

Honzig, M. P. 1976. Value and limitations of infant tests. In M. Lewis (Ed.), Origins of Intelligence. New York: Plenum Publishing Corp.

Hutt, C., and Ounsted, C. 1966. The biological significance of gaze aversion with particular reference to the syndrome of infantile autism. Behavioral Science, 11, 346–355.

Irwin, D. C., and Chen, H. P. 1946. Development of speech during infancy. Journal of Experimental Psychology, 36, 431–436.

Jerison, H. J. 1976. Paleoneurology and the evolution of mind. Scientific American, 234, 64–79.

Kanner, L. 1949. Problems of nosoiogy and psychodynamics of early infantile autism. American Journal of Orthopsychiatry, 19, 416–426.

Kazuk, E., Cohrs, M., and Frankenburg, W. K. 1974. Introduction to Pediatric Screening. Washington, D.C.: National Audiovisual Center, General Services Administration.

LADOCA Project. 1976. Denver Developmental Screening Test Kit, Manual, Score Pad. Denver.

Lenneberg, E. 1967. The Biological Foundation of Language. New York: John Wiley & Sons, Inc.

Lewis, M. 1976. Origins of Intelligence. New York: Plenum Publishing Corp.

Lewis, M., and Rosenblum, L. A. 1977. Interaction, Conversation, and the Development of Language. New York: John Wiley & Sons, Inc.

Loevinger, J. 1976. Ego Development. San Francisco: Jossey-Bass.

Lortie, D. C. 1975. School-teacher: A Sociological Study. Chicago: University of Chicago Press.

McLean, J. E., and Snyder-McLean, L. K. 1978. A Transactional Approach to Early Language Training. Columbus, Oh.: Charles E. Merrill Publishing Co.

McNeill, D. 1970. The development of language. In P. H. Mussen (Ed.), Carmichael's Manual of Child Psychology, Vol. 1. (3rd ed.). New York: John Wiley & Sons, Inc.

Marler, P. 1977. Sensory templates, vocal perception, and development: A comparative view. In M. Lewis and L. A. Rosenblum (Eds.), Interaction, Conversation and the Development of Language. New York: John Wiley & Sons, Inc.

Martin, B. 1975. Parent-child relations. In F. D. Horowitz (Ed.), Review of Child Development Research (Vol. 4). Chicago: University of Chicago Press.

Mercer, J. R. 1973. Labeling the Mentally Retarded. Berkeley: University of California Press.

Moerk, E. L. 1977. Pragmatic and Semantic Aspects of Early Language Development. Baltimore: University Park Press.

Neisser, U. 1967. Cognitive Psychology. New York: Appleton-Century-Crofts.

Neisser, U. 1976. Cognition and Reality. San Francisco: W. H. Freeman & Co.

Neligan, G., Prudham, D., and Steiner, H. 1974. Formative Years: Birth, Family and Development in Newcastle upon Tyne. London: Oxford University Press.

Nelson, K. 1973. Structure and strategy in learning to talk. Monographs of the society for research in child development, 38 (Serial No. 149).

Newman, B. M., and Newman, P. R. 1979. Development through Life: A Psychosocial Approach (Rev. ed.). Homewood, Ill.: The Dorsey Press.

Palermo, D. S., and Molfese, D. L. 1972. Language acquisition from age five onward. Psychological Bulletin, 73, 409-428.

Papousek, H. 1969. Individual variability in learner responses in human infants. In R. J. Robertson (Ed.), Brain and Early Behavior. London: Academic Press.

Piaget, J. 1970. Piaget's theory. In P. H. Mussen (Ed.), Carmichael's manual of child psychology. New York: John Wiley & Sons, Inc.

Piaget, J. 1971. Biology and Knowledge. Chicago: University of Chicago Press.

Richmond, J. B. 1975. An idea whose time has arrived. The Pediatric Clinics of North America, 22, 517-523.

Ricks, D. M. 1975. Vocal communication in pre-verbal normal and autistic children. In N. O'Connor (Ed.), Language, Cognitive Deficits, and Retardation. London: Butterworths.

Rimland, B. 1964. Infantile Autism. New York: Appleton-Century-Crofts.

Rossi, A. S. 1978. The biosocial side of parenthood. Human Nature, 1, 72-79.

Rovee, C. K., and Rovee, D. T. 1969. Conjugate reinforcement of infant exploratory behavior. Journal of Experimental Child Psychology, 8, 33-39.

Rudel, R. G. 1978. Neuroplasticity: Implications for development and education. In J. S. Chall and A. F. Mirsky (Eds.), Education and the Brain. Chicago: University of Chicago Press.

St. Clair, K. L. 1978. Neonatal assessment procedures: A historical review. Child Development, 49, 280-292.

Sameroff, A. J., and Chandler, M. J. 1975. Reproductive risk and the continuum of caretaking casualty. In F. D. Horowitz (Ed.), Review of Child Development Research (Vol. 4). Chicago: University of Chicago Press.

Scarr-Salapatek, S. 1975. Genetics and the development of intelligence. In F. D. Horowitz (Ed.), Review of Child Development Research (Vol. 4). Chicago: University of Chicago Press.

Scarr-Salapatek, S. 1976. An evolutionary perspective on infant intelligence: Species patterns and individual variations. In M. Lewis (Ed.), Origins of Intelligence. New York: Plenum Publishing Corp.

Spitz, R. A. 1945. Hospitalism: An inquiry into the genesis of psychiatric conditions in early childhood. Psychoanalytic Study of the Child, 1, 53-74.

Spitz, R. A. 1946. Anaclitic depression. Psychoanalytic Study of the Child, 2, 313-342.

Spock, B. 1957. Baby and Child Care. New York: Pocket Books.

Stein, Z. 1975. Review of Preschool IQ by S. H. Broman, P. L. Nichols, and W. A. Kennedy. Science, 188.

Stone, L. J., Smith, H. T., and Murphy, L. B. 1973. The Competent Infant. New York: Basic Books, Inc.

Teuber, H., and Rudel, R. G. 1962. Behavior after cerebral lesions in children and adults. Developmental Medicine and Child Neurology, 4, 3-20.

The Task Force on Pediatric Education. 1978. The Future of Pediatric Education. Evanston, Ill.: American Academy of Pediatrics.

Touwen, B. 1976. Neurological Development in Infancy. Philadelphia: J. B. Lippincott Co.

Ueda, R. 1978. Characteristics of child development in Okinawa: The comparisons with Tokyo and Denver and the implications for developmental screening. In W. K. Frankenburg (Ed.), Developmental Screening. Proceedings from the Second International Conference on Developmental Screening.

Vaillant, G. H. 1977. Adaptation to Life. Boston: Little, Brown & Company.

Werner, E. E., Bierman, J. M., and French, F. E. 1971. The Children of Kauai. Honolulu: University Press of Hawaii.

Werner, E. E., and Smith, R. S. 1977. Kauai's Children Come of Age. Honolulu: University Press of Hawaii.

Werner, H., and Kaplan, B. 1963. Symbol Formation. New York: John Wiley & Sons, Inc.

White, S. H. 1965. Evidence for a hierarchical arrangement of learning processes. In L. P. Lipsitt and C. C. Spiker (Eds.), Advances in Child Development and Behavior (Vol. 2). New York: Academic Press, Inc.

Wolff, P. H. 1969. The natural history of crying and other vocalizations in early infancy. In B. Foss (Ed.), Determinants of Infant Behavior (Vol. 4). London: Methuen.

Wulbert, M., Inglis, S., Kriegsman, E., and Mills, B. 1975. Language delay and associated mother-child interactions. Developmental Psychology, 2, 61–70.

Zelazo, P. R. 1972. Smiling and vocalizing: A cognitive emphasis. Merrill-Palmer Quarterly, 18, 349–367.

chapter **4**

AN APPROACH TO EXCEPTIONAL CHILDREN AND THEIR FAMILIES
Implications for Physician Education

Michael W. Yogman, William Sammons, and T. Berry Brazelton

How can medical school curricula be shaped to better prepare physicians to care for families with exceptional children? The answer to this question is twofold. The first part focuses on the care of these families — the way parents adjust when they realize that their child is exceptional, and the way physicians ensure access to and provide pediatric care for such children. In the second part of this chapter, the focus is on specific ways in which medical school educators can better train physicians to care for these families.

CARING FOR AN EXCEPTIONAL CHILD

The Grief Reaction

In caring for the families of exceptional children, one must first understand the concerns of the parents. When a baby is born with any impairment or illness, a parent's interactions with that child are dominated by a regular sequence of responses, which has been called a *grief reaction* (Drotar et al., 1975; Lindemann, 1944). For example, parents of a child with Down's syndrome will initially react with overwhelming shock characterized by much crying and feelings of hopelessness and helplessness.

Their expectations for a normal child have been violated, and they feel disappointed. At this point, the parents invariably blame themselves, wondering what they did wrong prior to, or during, the pregnancy. For example, a mother may be certain that her diet or unusual exercise were responsible. Such feelings of self-blame, inadequacy, and guilt are normal and expected, even though they often immobilize parents at this point. As the initial shock subsides, parents may try to handle their situation by denying the problem as if it were a bad dream. As the parents' denial and disbelief subside, they become increasingly angry and sad. Their anger may be directed at the baby, at themselves, and often at professionals such as pediatricians. Parents' anger at professionals can be understood as a projection of their anger at themselves and their perceived failure with their baby. Professionals may feel uncomfortable with the parents' denial and anger, and this discomfort can all too easily interfere with the supportive relationship that the parents need at this time. Parents may also delay their attachment to and isolate themselves from the baby, particularly if they are worried that the baby may die. The isolation and lack of attachment that may ensue are not from an absence of caring, but from caring too much. The blame that parents feel and the need to defend against that blame are intense and must be understood if one is to work with the parents.

So far, we have been describing the acute phase of parental grieving — a period of sadness and turmoil that is normal and expected and that every parent of an exceptional child is likely to experience to some degree. These reactions can easily be misinterpreted to imply parental pathology. During this acute period, the pediatrician can play a supportive and empathic role, providing understanding for parents' expressions of their feelings (that it is okay to feel sad or angry), while, at the same time, offering and clarifying information about the baby's problems.

As parents adapt, they begin to feel less anxious and are more comfortable caring for their babies. Because the timing of this shift is highly variable, it represents a transition to a more chronic stage of grieving in which parents can give up the more expensive defenses of denial and projection and free themselves for the real work that they must accomplish with their child. By being available and recognizing when parents are ready to work, the pediatrician can play a very useful role in answering the family's questions, in helping the parents recognize the baby's strengths without denying the deficits, and in helping the parents avoid treating the baby as more vulnerable than necessary.

These two stages of acute and chronic parental grieving illustrate the way parents, with appropriate supports, can transform their own reactions from ones that seem at first to interfere with the child's development to ones that optimize it.

In most families, parental feelings and reactions, similar to the ones experienced initially, may periodically recur. Often this occurs at times when the parent's expectations for the child to achieve a normal developmental milestone are disappointed. For example, the social smile in infants with Down's syndrome appears at the usual time, 2 months, but it lacks the full facial and visual brightening present in other infants. Parents of these babies are very disappointed at this time, almost as much as they were when they first learned about the baby's problem (Emde and Brown, 1978). At such times, a physician can help the parents understand what triggered the recurrence of these feelings, deal with their own disappointment, and reinforce the child's positive self-image and sense of competence.

In partial summary, a major thesis of this chapter is that although early interactions between parents and handicapped children appear different, such reactions by parents are expected and are the first stage of the process of adaptation in which parents refocus their energies. The job of professionals is to back parents up so that they are better able to continue the process of negotiation with their child, searching for the strengths and adaptations within each of them that will optimize the child's later development.

Evaluation and Assessment

If one now considers the needs of the children for pediatric care, almost all of these children require evaluation and assessment. Frequently, medicine translates this need into an energetic search for an immediate and unitary diagnosis with a single etiology. Some children may require and may benefit immediately from the establishment of such a firm diagnosis, particularly where it implies a single, straightforward treatment. But the exhaustive and exclusive search for a single diagnosis may be costly and inappropriate for many problems and may displace a more comprehensive assessment of the child's needs. Often, multiple factors are involved in the genesis of these problems and, almost always, emotional and social components, as well as biological components, are essential to the clinical science of providing effective management. It seems useful here to emphasize the distinction between a one-shot diagnosis and repeated assessments that, by documenting change over time, are likely to be more predictive of later function.

All too often, professionals focus exclusively on the child's difficulties and fail to consider the areas in which the child functions well. A better understanding of the way in which the processes of normal development are influenced by a given handicap is necessary to reverse this emphasis. An understanding of the processes of normal development includes the child's adaptations, coping mechanisms, styles, and competencies, as well as any deficits. A comprehensive assessment can substitute a profile of the child's functions — his/her areas of strength and of weakness — for an often meaningless diagnostic label. This assessment should include an in-depth look at specific areas of neuromotor, cognitive, perceptual, temperamental, language, and social-emotional development, as well as the integration of all these developmental processes. By considering the child's influence on the environment in each of these areas and the reciprocal influence of the environment on the child, one is better able to pinpoint the child's needs and his/her ways of meeting those needs.

Identification of the child's strengths is a powerful reinforcer for the child's own internal coping and adaptive capacities. The self-fulfilling prophecy or expectancy effect is a powerful one, as documented in *Pygmalion in the Classroom* (Rosenthal and Jacobson, 1968). By consciously looking for strengths, one may even use the expectancy effect as an intervention. Models for coping and adaptation now exist that delineate the way life stresses or adversity, when combined with appropriate support, can lead to healthy adaptation. Frequently, these models are forgotten when dealing with exceptional children, particularly where the only assessments used are those that document deficits, e.g., the milestones the child has not achieved. One of the real needs in medicine is the need for better instruments to assess the strengths and coping of children, particularly those with handicaps. The goal of professionals in working with these families should be to maximize the functional competence of the individual child and the adaptation of the family. This goal is often forgotten, and instead, more arbitrary goals are substituted, based on wishes that a child perform according to some idealized expectations — a course that often leads to frustration and disappointment of both professionals and parents.

Although this section has addressed the care of families who have ready access to health care, unfortunately a ready access to health care is often not the case for all families (Children's Defense Fund, 1978). In assuming responsibility for the health care of children, physicians, together with other professionals, need to play a more important role in reaching out to families and in ensuring that all exceptional children receive the comprehensive assessments and management they deserve.

Clinician-Family Relationships

At this point, one might ask how a clinician can work with the exceptional child and his/her parents with the goals of maximizing functional competence and family adaptation. The first step is consciously working to develop a relationship with the parents, which can be characterized as one of mutual — participation or guidance — cooperation, rather than an active

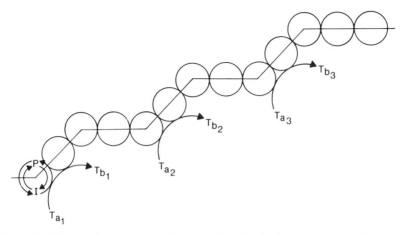

Figure 1. Touch points for intervention. A schematic developmental curve of parent-infant interaction (P-I) with treatment interventions (Ta → Tb) superimposed at certain sensitive times (1, 2, 3).

doctor and a passive parent (Szasz and Hollender, 1956). In order to develop this relationship, the pediatrician must be able to use and understand his/her own feelings as important clinical data that serve as a guide to where he/she is in the development of a relationship. In this manner, the recognition and management of problems need not be overwhelming to either doctor or parent; parents can feel comfortable openly exploring their deeper concerns and fears and freely describing and searching for the supports and resources they need, without feeling ashamed or apologetic. Second, clinical intervention is most effective when it can be individualized and be appropriate to the child's level of development. It is important to realize that there are discontinuities in development, periods of organization and disorganization within the broader child-environment system (see Chapter 3, this volume). Intervention need not and probably should not be continuous, but it should be sensitive to periods of disorganization and times of particular vulnerability, such as the disorganization that occurs when a baby with Down's syndrome is 2 months old (Emde and Brown, 1978). Figure 1 shows schematically sensitive times, or touch points, for intervention superimposed on a developmental curve of spurts and plateaus. Certain times when new developmental skills appear or are anticipated (the spurts on the curve) represent important touch points for intervention when the system is more open to change.

Articulating the baby's behavior with parents of exceptional children seems particularly important. Discussions of the specifics of the child's development and behavior can be a way of promoting the parent's acceptance of their baby as an individual. It allows the pediatrician to communicate with parents in a nonthreatening manner, because both the pediatrician and the parents can see the same behavior. Furthermore, being able to anticipate developmental issues for the child and the parent has implications for prevention of later problems. The technique is illustrated by the study of an infant who is blind from birth. A videotape was used to film interactions between the baby and the parents so that the tapes could be replayed and the baby's behavior could be discussed with the parents (Als, 1977). Viewing the tapes allowed the parents to see and to describe for themselves how they were encouraging the child's autonomy.

SHAPING THE MEDICAL SCHOOL CURRICULUM

How can these ideas be integrated into the medical school curriculum? First, it seems critical to emphasize the importance of the institutional commitment by the medical school and of the personal commitment by senior faculty to the value of physicians becoming child and family advocates and experts on "the whole child," not just on individual organ systems. Any teaching program will encounter great difficulties without a sympathetic value structure reflected throughout the institution.

To a great extent, the broad needs of exceptional children are best met by a training program that addresses similar issues in all children — understanding people's strengths, the processes of adaptation, and the way people use relationships. In part, this program requires a return to the skills of the old-fashioned clinician whose diagnostic armamentarium was more limited to his eyes, hands, and ears, and less dependent on instrumentation. The difference now is that medical education requires a new synthesis of increasing amounts of technical knowledge, along with the clinical skills of learning to look and to listen, in order to elicit clinical data and to establish and use relationships so that patients can benefit from the technical knowledge.

A modified medical record seems to be a useful method of teaching that facilitates this synthesis. In most schools, medical students are now taught to use the problem-oriented system of medical record keeping (Weed, 1969), a system that easily lends itself to clinical teaching. Certain modifications make this method of medical record keeping even more useful to physicians caring for children. In contrast to listing only the problems a child or patient may have (familial and perinatal risk factors, physical anomalies, neurological findings), the student simultaneously records in a parallel fashion the strengths that the child and the family demonstrate — particularly those strengths evidenced by coping strategies and the availability of social supports. Just as this record of problems and strengths evolves as the child develops, the student also specifies the nature of the relationship he/she is establishing with the parent as that relationship develops. This record emphasizes the fact that the quality and level of the doctor-parent-child relationship influences the kind of data about problems and strengths that a parent may feel comfortable discussing with a physician. Students are thus led to conclude that improving their relationship with a parent may be the crucial first step toward obtaining the data necessary for either diagnosis or management. For example, the student may realize that a relationship based on mutual participation is more helpful for managing a problem than an active-passive relationship. At the end of each encounter, the student is asked to record explicit goals for parent and child — short-term goals for the next visit, and long-term goals as well. These goals may involve such areas as: fostering the parent's ability to encourage the child's autonomy, or encouraging the parent to describe the child's behavior in a way that allows optimal, efficient pediatric care in managing acute illnesses, behavioral problems, or health maintenance. A sample of this kind of medical record keeping form used with the family of a high risk premature infant is shown in Table 1. The form acknowledges the importance of the doctor-parent relationship, patient strengths as well as problems, and goal setting by the physician. Its value to students is that it forces them to make explicit the data behind the intuitions that guide so much of clinical medicine.

Just as this form of medical record keeping helps students think about the development of their relationships with a patient, medical school educators need to pay more attention to the students' development into professional physicians. The manner in which students grapple with such issues as caring for chronically ill patients, feeling responsible for a patient's care, and identifying with a patient are all critical to the development of defenses that can either be adaptive or maladaptive for both students and their patients, especially exceptional children. For example, caring for a handicapped child can generate feelings of one's own vulnerability — that there but for fate go I. As students become more aware of how their own reactions to these children influence their care, they may be able to find alternatives to avoiding or fleeing from these children. The issue is heightened if students have their own children. In this case, students may struggle between extremes — either overidentifying with the parents or dehumanizing the family — unless they understand their reactions and find alternative role models for an "empathic identification" with the family, which allows the students to maintain both their humanity and identity. As the students assume increasing responsibility for the care of patients, they grapple with an unrealistic sense of their omnipotence, expecting to cure everyone if only they knew the right answer. Opportunities for students to express their feelings about this awesome responsibility may help the student give up the defense of abandoning the exceptional child that one cannot cure or of focusing only on a single

Table 1. Sample medical record keeping form

	Data Base			Goals	
Relationship	Strengths	Problems	Short-term		Long-term
1. Initial meeting, mother distant and passive, avoids eye contact	Mother: high school graduate with career aspirations	Mother: adolescent, unplanned pregnancy Infant: premature	Developing trust		
2. Became more animated (smiled) when M.D. recalled mother's observations at previous visit	Baby discharged at 2 weeks, mother roomed in on final hospital day	Family history of mental retardation	Assessing infant's physical and psychological status		
3. More quickly came to talk animatedly about her concerns	Played lovingly with baby, appropriate handling of baby	Difficult to bring baby to alert state	Develop individualized relationship with mother		Establish mutual goals with parent that encompass areas of health maintenance and development
4. Father accompanies mother at this visit	Strong family supports, involved father		Assessing baby's development and using it to support mother		
5. Mother asks frequent questions, shares feelings, transactional relationship	Infant socially responsive		Discuss infant's progress, behavior and development, individuality, and giving mother feeling of having reached a goal		Facilitate parental acceptance of infant's developmental changes, i.e. increasing autonomy

organ system. A physician caring for exceptional children must be able to tolerate a degree of uncertainty about the prognosis and must help parents do the same. A sense of one's own limits, as well as one's authentic responsibilities, seems a critical and yet much neglected aspect of professional training, particularly for physicians working with parents of exceptional children who may show denial or who project anger to the physician. At several medical schools, educators have attempted to accomplish these goals by providing tutorials and support groups for students from the first year on as part of a course in physical diagnosis (Werner and Korsch, 1976).

Incorporating Critical Concepts: The First Two Years

As this point, an analogy between the development of a physician in medical school and developmental processes in other aspects of life seems warranted. During the four years of medical school there are periods when students are optimally available and eager to learn about caring for the broad needs of children.

The first two years of medical school are often times of delayed gratification. Most students enter school full of enthusiasm about caring for people, but instead are faced with a barrage of knowledge, books, and competition from peers. As the amount of medical knowledge continues to expand, there are increasingly competitive demands for course time, and although little can be added to the curriculum, the way in which material is presented can be changed. For example, the presentation of patients in basic science classes can be done much more effectively. A parent enters carrying a child with myelomeningocele. The professor asks if anyone has any questions, and there is a painful silence. Most students understand the embryology, but they know little else about the problem. It is difficult for them to relate it to that time, still two years away, when they start to care for patients. The professors need to describe how the family became attached to and grieved about the baby, how they decided about surgery, how they dealt with difficult ethical questions, and why coping with that problem was so difficult. The students would then have some questions to ask. They would be back in touch with the patient.

The opportunities for changing the methods of presentation of the curriculum materials are unlimited. Down's syndrome is often discussed during genetics classes. The study of genetics often considers all the statistics, but it would be more exciting to show a tape of or playact a scene of genetic counseling.

Psychiatry can also take a different approach. It may be interesting to talk about such issues as transference/countertransference in terms of hospital admissions, as well as abstract lecture concepts. The grief reaction need not only focus on death and dying, but it also needs to be understood as it occurs in parents of handicapped children. Many schools do not even formally consider death and dying until the student/house officer is faced with a dying patient — and then he/she is often very alone.

Other schools have tried to give the first year medical student a practical education in patient relationship formation by having him/her follow a patient. Although this model is expensive in terms of preceptor time, it offers the student a unique exposure to a continuous relationship with a family in which the student can understand the adjustments and adaptations that families make on a day-to-day basis. With proper support, it can be a remarkable experience where the student has the opportunity to understand many different levels of patient relationships and coping, as well as disease. In fact, following a patient offers one answer to the peculiarities of training in which students are exposed mainly to acute episodes on a short-term basis, while physicians in practice spend most of their time helping patients deal with the chronic aspects of their illness or disability (Korsch, 1976).

During the second year, the student feels a combination of elation and terror as he/she anticipates caring for patients. The challenge is at two levels: 1) cognitively, what do I know and how will I learn all the other information, and 2) establishing a fulfilling relationship with the patients.

Mechanistically, the easiest way to teach students about the relationship is during the physical diagnosis course. The first class is usually spent extolling the importance of a "good history," for example, statements such as the "history is 90% of the diagnosis" are familiar. Why then is over 90% of the remaining time in the course spent on learning the physical exam? The well-known work of Korsch (Korsch, 1956; Korsch and Negrete, 1972) documents how much can be taught about interviewing and developing a relationship with parents. When the interview is seen as therapeutic as well as diagnostic, it becomes used for more than fact gathering and a standard review of systems. Students need to see that the quality of their relationship with a patient influences the quality of the history they can elicit. They need to view the interview in terms of the relationship they are establishing with that patient. How does the student feel about what he/she is doing? A student's feelings about death and the examination of the other sex probably influence the patient's feelings. The student needs to learn more about himself/herself and the patient at the same time, since the way a student feels about a patient may not only affect what history is obtained, but the student's gut reactions may become the best measure of the patient's progress.

The Third Year

During the third year, most medical schools provide close personal supervision during clinical rotations. As a model of the physician-patient relationship, the preceptors need to see the student's strengths as well as difficulties when making rounds, observing an examination, or correcting write-ups. Much of this can be done on an individual level, but students can learn much from each other about patient relationships if they meet regularly as a group. There is a certain camaraderie as all students enter this new phase, and small ad hoc groups naturally form among students on the same rotation. During this period, the student often feels very concerned about his/her competence — he/she is at the bottom of the totem pole, cannot start IVs, and hardly knows anything about congestive heart failure. By working in parallel on relationship formation, preceptors can foster positive feelings of success at a time when those feelings are desperately wanted, and also at an important stage of developing that individual's doctor-patient relationship style. Viewed in these terms, the interview becomes not only a challenge to develop new skills, but it also can serve as a balancing factor to relieve many other feelings about failure. Almost all students are willing to invest a lot of energy in knowing the patient for their own personal reasons because feedback from the patient is usually positive and reinforces that relationship.

Furthermore, the hospital staff puts a certain premium on the role of the medical student because he/she is the one person on ward rounds who is acknowledged to know something more about the patient than just the barest personal history and the medical facts. Often the resident or the attending physician feels that there is some importance in the patient's "social history" that he cannot articulate. In response, the student often starts a nonselective recitation — and somebody stops him saying, "Get to the point." Often this occurs because the student's history is centered around problems, not around strengths. Therefore, the student's recitation rarely helps in the management of the patient, but it is just one more item on the list of complications. There is no feeling that a recitation will really help, and often the problems are shunted to someone else — welfare for example — and the patient feels shunted at the same time. The student needs to be explicit about the patient's strengths and about the way stress can produce positive changes. Rather than talking about the difficult adolescent or the hostile parent, different information is conveyed by stating how a parent is coping with grieving over a child's handicaps. There is always some developmental process, and this information needs to be framed that way — a fever is always put in context, why not the tears as well?

Certainly the model discussed so far is generalizable to the surgeon as well as the pediatrician, at least theoretically. By the end of the third year, the student who has decided to go into pediatrics is often taking a number of electives. As a doctor he/she has learned a great deal about himself/herself and about adults, and now he/she is ready to learn more about children. A pediatric clerkship/elective can offer the opportunity to learn about children — their ability to excite, their resilience, their developmental stages — the teasing 18-month-old and the hesitant 4-year-old.

Importance of Direct Observations in Typical Settings Given the difficulties of learning about the normal range of children's behavior (in particular their strengths) in a hospital or clinic setting, it is not surprising that students dramatically improve their understanding of children by observing them in such settings as schools and day care centers. Students realize that they can describe children's behavior and their own feelings in a way that is reliable and no longer seems "soft." These experiences allow students to gain a fundamental understanding of key concepts, such as attachment and separation; coping; the importance of understanding children as individuals; mastery, competence, and self-esteem as driving forces in development; and the fact that adults have their own feelings when working with children. All of these concepts are crucial for understanding the exceptional child, particularly since professionals need to work together in teams in caring for these children. These experiences also allow students to see the powerful influences of peer interactions on a child as well as the influences of community settings and the implications of political decision-making on child care. In addition, the adults are no longer patients, they are parents. The student is faced with forming two different relationships — one with the parents and one with the child. He/she can certainly build on the previously evolving skills, but this is a time when the student needs a different kind of support to move beyond understanding relationships with parents to think in terms of coping strategies and the developmental organization of children.

These experiences also form a base for teaching students techniques for assessing development. They encourage the student to recognize the complexity of development and the need for a conceptual base to evaluate and use assessment techniques as they are modified by new research. If students have a conceptual framework as a base, they are much less likely to misuse assessment techniques. Especially for exceptional children, the student needs to be able to use assessments to better understand the way developmental issues shape the concerns at a family level, including the concerns of parents and siblings (Pless and Pinkerton, 1975). For example, if a student is seeing a family with a 2-year-old child with a handicap, his/her pediatric goals must attend to the way the family unit is negotiating the child's independence and autonomy.

Looking at the patient relationships in this manner is exciting because it reflects many of the reasons why people choose to be pediatricians. The exuberance of new discoveries and the honesty and spontaneity of children fuel all pediatric relationships.

A seminar on the developmental implications of handicaps might become an ongoing study group for those going into pediatrics. It will take a long time to work out all the aspects of telling a child/parent that he/she will never walk again. What does a pediatrician say to the new mother whose child is deaf or blind? What does a pediatrician say to the parent whose only son, 6-months old, has severe meningitis when he/she is not sure what the long-range outcome will be? Obviously, students on other rotations (infectious disease, neonatology, surgery) could continue to participate in this seminar.

The Fourth Year

By the final years of medical school, the student's identity as a physician has solidified enough so that it is a good time to focus on how professionals work together in teams. Students are now eager to contrast the concerns and the problems in the acute diagnostic phase with the ongoing follow-up relationship. The acute grieving is not the same as the chronic process for the patient, for the doctor, or for the parents. The fourth year student has usually started to develop a feeling for "my patient," which drives him/her to care not only about the acute diagnostic process, but also about the follow-up of the patient. In many ways this is the culmination of the medical school experience, and the coalescence of a true psychosomatic model. Now the student can see other types of developmental stages, he/she can really learn about chronic grieving and adjustment, and he/she can learn about preventive medicine — at both the organic and affective level.

This kind of teaching model can restore to medical school training the idealism and the importance of working with people that the students have when they enroll. As students leave medical school they would be better prepared to work with the special needs of exceptional children and their families as well as with the strengths and weaknesses that all families have. They would be better able to recognize the strength and the value of the individuality and diversity of all children — that in fact all children are exceptional in their own way. And finally, they would quickly realize how much more they can do for exceptional children if they are willing to help the members of their families with their feelings.

REFERENCES

Als, H. 1977. Affective reciprocity and the development of autonomy: The study of a blind infant. Paper presented to Society for Research in Child Development, New Orleans.
Children's Defense Fund. 1978. EPSDT in Practice: What's happening in the field? American Journal of Orthopsychiatry, 48, 77–95.

Drotar, D., Baskiewicz, A., Irwin, N., Kennell, J., and Klaus, M. 1975. The Adaptation of parents to the birth of an infant with a congenital malformation: A hypothetical model. Pediatrics, 56, 710–717.

Emde, R., and Brown, C. 1978. Adaptation to the birth of a Down's syndrome infant. Journal of the American Academy Child Psychiatry, 17, 299–323.

Korsch, B. 1956. Practical techniques of observing interviewing and advising parents in pediatric practice as demonstrated in an attitude study project. Pediatrics 18, 467–490.

Korsch, B. 1976. Chronic illness in childhood and family functions. In V. Vaughan and T. B. Brazelton (Eds.), The Family: Can It Be Saved? Chicago: Year Book Medical Publishers, Inc.

Korsch, B., and Negrete, V. F. 1972. Doctor-patient communication. Scientific American 227, 66–74.

Lindemann, E. 1944. Symptomatology and management of acute grief. American Journal of Psychiatry 101, 141–148.

Pless, I. B., and Pinkerton, P. 1975. Chronic Childhood Disorder: Promoting Patterns of Adjustment, Chicago: Year Book Medical Publishers, Inc.

Rosenthal, R., and Jacobson, L. 1968. Pygmalion in the Classroom: Teacher Expectation and Pupils' Intellectual Development. New York: Holt, Rinehart & Winston, Inc.

Szasz, T., and Hollender, M. 1956. A contribution to the philosophy of medicine: The basic models of the doctor patient relationship. Archives of Internal Medicine, 97, 585–592.

Weed, L. L. 1969. Medical Records, Medical Education and Patient Care: The Problem Oriented Medical Record. Cleveland: The Press of Case Western Reserve University.

Werner, E. R., and Korsch, B. 1976. The vulnerability of the medical student: Posthumous presentation of L. L. Stephens' ideas. Pediatrics 57, 321–328.

chapter 5

A FRAMEWORK FOR CURRICULUM DESIGN

Michael S. Levine

The Learning Unit consists of the learner, the learning resources (teacher and materials), and the curriculum. This chapter focuses on one part of the Learning Unit, the curriculum. A curriculum guides the interactions between the learner and the learning resources. It is the teacher's communication to students about where they are going, how they will get there, and how they will know when they have arrived. The curriculum is a learning map. A curriculum must have its parts clearly related to each other and it must be arranged to ensure economical, orderly learning. A curriculum for physician training about exceptional children must identify the general attitudes, cognitive resources, and psychomotor skills that the physician will require in practice. The specific learning objectives, the learning activities, and the standards of performance are then derived from these general statements. Both the learner and the teacher should be familiar with the entire learning map (Stritter and Talbert, 1974).

PROBLEMS IN PHYSICIAN EDUCATION

Unfortunately, the curriculum in most training programs in medicine is characterized by serendipity and idiosyncrasy. The learner spends an arbitrary amount of time in a training setting, hoping, through brownian movement, to encounter the common and enough of the uncommon problems in the area to be a successful practitioner. But this encounter is not really random because the clinical problems that present themselves are idiosyncratically skewed by the interests of the teacher and the reputation of the training center. Inevitably this approach results in a striking lack of correspondence between the learning experience and actual practice (Kane, Woolley, and Kane, 1973).

Randomness and lack of relevance are not the only problems with physician education. Traditionally, the emphasis has been on the acquisition of factual information (Dudley, 1970; Weed, 1976). Unfortunately, facts are both forgotten and outdated quickly. If a supply of facts is a physician's major resource, he/she is quickly left with nothing to assist his/her patients. Many medical educators now believe that we should develop other strengths in the learners, such as the powers of decision-making (Schwartz et al., 1973), logical reasoning, reliability, thoroughness (Weed, 1976), and the development of appropriate attitudes toward patient care (Helder, Verbrugh, and de Vries, 1977). These intellectual skills will always be useful, allowing the physician to remain relevant. However, these suggestions have been mostly ignored in actual learning settings and almost totally ignored in the evaluation of learners.

Another problem with medical education is that it often mismatches the complexity of the task with the level of competence of the trainee. Furthermore, the activities at various levels of competence are not sequentially related. When learning activities are not ordered according to difficulty and do not take into consideration the readiness state of the learner, the novice is bewildered by complexity and the advanced student is bored. However, with forethought, one can relate all levels of training and can structure a training program of progressively more complex tasks.

NEW APPROACHES TO CURRICULUM DESIGN

Research in the field of learning in the last 20 years has begun to clarify learning activities. One advance is the assignment of learning activities to either an affective, cognitive, or psychomotor domain (Dressel, 1976). This advance allows us to order and identify the activities of the students, which is the first step in ending random learning. This analysis is now being applied to medical education (Kane, Woolley, and Kane, 1973). Another advance is the recognition that educational objectives must be clearly defined. The absence of defined objectives is cited as the first ranking deficiency in British medical education (*Goals and Objectives in Medical Education,* 1977). Broad statements of intent (goals) lead to precise statements of what the student must do (objectives). Developing procedures for defining objectives has become a major field of study in itself (*Objectives in Medical Education,* 1977).

Training physicians to care for exceptional children must not be done in a manner that recapitulates the errors of general medical education. The basic curriculum that follows was developed to overcome these deficiencies. Its five goals are:

1. To assure comprehensive coverage of the skills and knowledge necessary to evaluate and remediate the problems of exceptional children by rational and conscious selection of subject matter.
2. To assist the learner to develop in himself/herself the necessary skills of sound analysis, accurate data gathering, responsibility, thoroughness, compassion, and self-awareness.
3. To bind together acquisition of skills and knowledge about the patient and promotion of personal growth in the learner within a single curriculum.
4. To provide a basic curriculum that can be easily concretized by construction of specific educational objectives and learning activities by the teacher who will use it.
5. To facilitate the creation of particularized curricula at all levels of training that are logically related.

THE BASIC CURRICULUM

The conceptual framework of the basic curriculum is based coequally on the patient and the learner. The unifying concepts of the curriculum are comprehensiveness and integration. Evaluation and treatment planning must be comprehensive because exceptional children often have multiple problems, all of which must be dealt with if one expects a successful outcome. Integration of these patient-oriented activities with trainee-oriented learning is required if we are to produce competent, self-knowledgeable practitioners.

In this basic curriculum, learning for physicians-in-training is arranged in a hierarchy from general topics to specific topics (Figure 1). Factual knowledge and the ability to solve problems are learned in relation to three organizing concepts: the child (Figure 2), the family (Figure 3), and society (Figure 4). Knowledge of the child, the family, and society are the three concentric loci of dysfunction relevant to the exceptional child. They all must be included in comprehensive evaluation and treatment; therefore they are basic to the curriculum. The relationship between items is clearly developed in a deductive fashion. The particularized curriculum is then derived from the basic curriculum. The particularized curriculum is to be constructed by the teacher who will use it and therefore is only generally described here.

The trainee's learning is related to the organizing concepts (child, family, or society) according to the domain of learning involved (cognitive, affective, or psychomotor) (see Figure 1). Placing all subjects into one of these categories is a useful, proven method of organizing learning activities. These domains are subdivided into levels, with patient-centered and learner-centered subjects distinctly identified, but indivisibly linked.

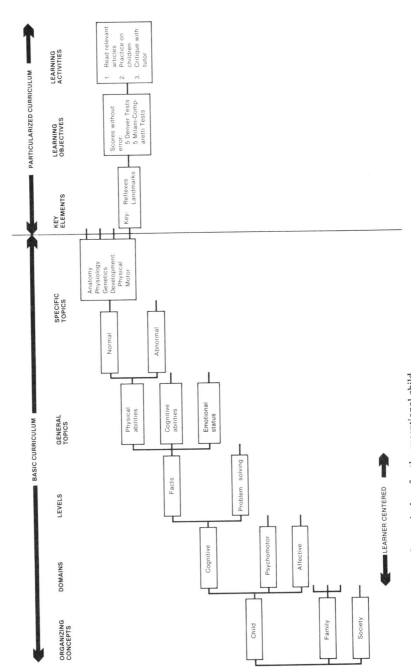

Figure 1. Overview of a curriculum for the exceptional child.

The patient-centered subject matter follows within the appropriate learning domain, first organized by general topics and then subdivided into specific topics. It is at the level of specific topics that traditional curriculum planning often begins (cf., Richardson, Guralnick, and Tupper, 1978). The specific topics are the most concrete statements possible for a curriculum of general applicability. They clearly indicate the breadth and depth required to educate competent physicians in this field. Yet, they are not so concrete that the teacher using the basic curriculum cannot tailor it to suit his/her overall course goals, available resources, and trainees' readiness.

Particularized Curriculum: The Teacher's Task

The basic curriculum can be used to structure medical student or resident training programs in pediatric habilitation by deriving different particularized curriculums. The teacher who uses the basic curriculum particularizes it by identifying more narrowly defined subjects, herein called elements, logically derived from the specific topics of the basic curriculum. The teacher must make a conscious decision in selecting elements for the particularized curriculum. In a holistic learning environment, this selection is done by the student and the teacher together. They then develop specific measurable learning objectives. These objectives state precisely what behavior the learner will exhibit at the end and how it will be measured. (For example, "The trainee will complete five *Denver Developmental* evaluations on five different children, recording the results. He/she will make no more than one error on each exam when his/her scoring is compared to that of an observer scoring the same exam.") Finally, the teacher will arrange learning activities through which the objectives will be reached. (Examples of learning activities could include patient evaluation, discussions with the instructor, programmed or standard texts, oral presentation of a topic, setting up and carrying out a research project, or supervising less experienced learners.) The selection of learning activities and objectives will depend on the student's readiness and available time, on the number of learners at any one time, on the teacher's educational philosophy and course objectives, and on the learning materials and clinical opportunities available.

IMPLICATIONS AND CONCLUSIONS

The use of this basic curriculum to structure specific course development will ensure comprehensive, integrated, rational educational planning. All important patient-related topics are included. Learner-oriented activities are prominent and explicit. The interrelationship between patient topics and learner topics is clear. Idiosyncratic exposure to material is minimized

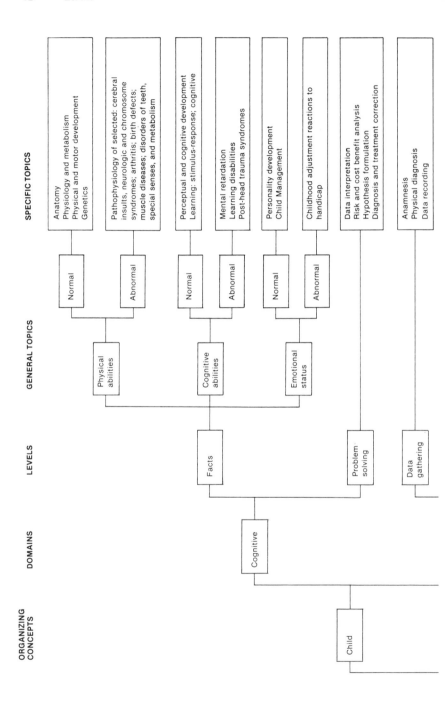

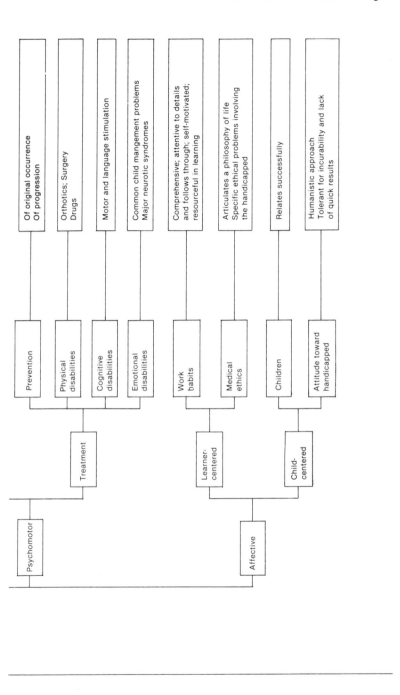

Figure 2. Curriculum structure through the organizing concept of the child.

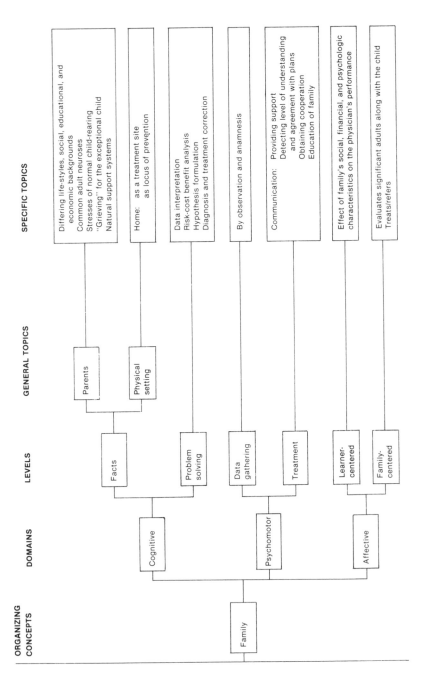

Figure 3.   Curriculum structure through the organizing concept of the family.

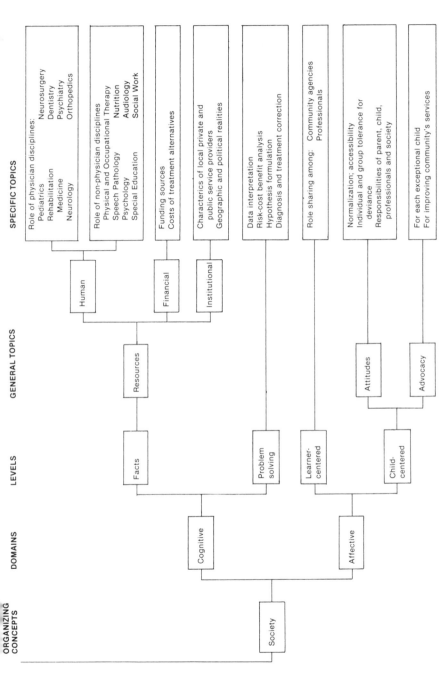

Figure 4.   Curriculum structure through the organizing concept of society.

because any changes will be made after consciously weighing the alternatives. Teacher planning energy can therefore be directed toward selecting a detailed particularized curriculum and to student and course evaluation.

A particularized curriculum allows students to know what skills and attributes they are expected to exhibit at the completion of the training program and how they are expected to acquire them. This will reduce the bewilderment of the novice learner by providing rational boundaries to the tasks. Elements and learning activities can be easily isolated and varied experimentally to improve learning. Biases in program coverage will be easy to detect. Finally, the basic curriculum provides a structure to use in comparing the content and emphasis of different training programs.

REFERENCES

Dressel, P. L. 1976. Handbook of Academic Evaluation. San Francisco: Jossey-Bass.
Dudley, H. A. F. 1970. Taxonomy of clinical educational objectives. British Journal of Medical Education, 4, 13–18.
Goals and Objectives in Medical Education: An Editorial. 1977. The Lancet, 1, 985–986.
Helder, H., Verbrugh, H. S., and de Vries, M. J. 1977. Toward an holistic education in pathology and medicine. Journal of Medical Education, 52, 648–653.
Kane, R., Woolley, F. R., and Kane, R. 1973. Toward defining the end product of medical education. Journal of Medical Education, 48, 615–624.
Objectives in Medical Education: An Editorial. 1977. British Journal of Medical Education, 11, 241–243.
Richardson, H. B., Guralnick, M. J., and Tupper, D. B. 1978. Training pediatricians for effective involvement with handicapped preschool children and their families. Mental Retardation, 16, 3–7.
Schwartz, W. B., Gorry, G. A., Kassirer, J. P., and Essig, A. 1973. Decision analysis and clinical judgment. The American Journal of Medicine, 55, 459–472.
Stritter, F. T., and Talbert, L. M. 1974. An empirical approach to instruction in obstetrics and gynecology. Journal of Medical Education, 49, 770–777.
Weed, L. L. 1976. A new paradigm for medical education. In E. S. Purcell (Ed.), Recent Trends in Medical Education. New York: Josiah Macey, Jr. Foundation.

chapter 6

EVALUATING COMPETENCIES
Relationship to Content of a Developmental Disabilities Curriculum for Physicians

Victor C. Vaughan, III

In 1972, the American Board of Pediatrics (ABP) undertook a study aimed at making more explicit and relevant the relationship between the content of its examinations in pediatrics and the competencies that it felt physicians should have in order to be certified as pediatricians. The Board appointed a number of task forces composed of practicing pediatricians and pediatric educators and charged them with defining and displaying the competencies of pediatricians.

These task forces set about their business with zeal. It soon became apparent that the number of discrete items that were thought appropriate for the competency of pediatricians was becoming so large that their compilation could result only in a document of mammoth and unwieldy size. The Board found itself in a predicament analogous to that of a medical school that some years ago attempted to catalog all the items of knowledge and technical skill that a medical student should master before receiving a medical degree. After a year or two of compiling items that were believed to be essential for the armamentarium of the physician, approximately one-quarter million items had been collected, and these represented approximately one-half of the total that would be required. It can be calculated that if a medical student were to incorporate all the items at a rate of one item every 2 minutes, 12 hours a day, 7 days a week, 48 weeks a year, for each of 4 years of medical school, the student would fail by more than 6 weeks to complete the assigned task.

THE ORGANIZATION OF COMPETENCIES

At this point, the Board changed tactics and undertook an analysis of the competencies that had been identified in order to see what general features the competencies had that could assist in the development of a relevant evaluation program. The result was the definition of certain *abilities,* which were important for the pediatrician, and certain *tasks,* which were to embrace what a pediatrician is ordinarily called upon to do with these abilities. The abilities and tasks were then set against each other in the form of a matrix (Figure 1) (American Board of Pediatrics, Inc., 1974; Burg et al., 1976).

The matrix sets five abilities (*attitudes, factual knowledge, interpersonal skills, technical skills,* and *clinical judgment*) against three tasks, (*gathering, organizing, and recording data; assessing data;* and *managing problems and maintaining health*). To each of the 15 cells of the matrix, a number of statements can be assigned with regard to competencies generally required of pediatricians; moreover, if the concept embodied by the matrix is applied to a specific medical problem, such as meningitis, the contents of the various cells can be made highly specific to the problem presented. Figure 2 presents one such application of this model.

This matrix has proved to be a powerful tool, not only for evaluation, but for education as well. It has given us a way of parsing a great variety of clinical problems into those features that are appropriate for evaluation, and it displays those features in a way that makes it easier to choose the features that have high priority and those that have low priority.

The matrix has helped those who develop the Board's examinations to achieve, in specific content areas, a concept that has increasingly been considered to be important by educators, in and out of medicine: that the goals of both education and evaluation be made more relevant and that they be more consistent with each other.

The ABP has long been aware that its written and oral examinations are substantially limited as to how much of the universe of competencies they can sample. In the areas of attitudes and technical skills, for example, relatively little can be learned with confidence from the traditional certifying examinations. Factual knowledge can be assessed with a high degree of reliability, and some impressions can be gained with regard to interpersonal skills and clinical judgments; but the Board has thought it necessary to rely heavily upon the directors of training programs to supply essential information regarding the preparedness of pediatricians in the other areas.

Abilities	Tasks		
	1—Gathering, organizing and recording data	2—Assessing data	3—Managing problems and maintaining health
A—Attitudes	A1	A2	A3
B—Factual knowledge	B1	B2	B3
C—Interpersonal skills	C1	C2	C3
D—Technical skills	D1	D2	D3
E—Clinical judgment	E1	E2	E3

Figure 1.   Matrix associating tasks and abilities. (Reprinted by permission from the American Board of Pediatrics, Inc., 1974.)

Tasks

Abilities	1—Gathering, organizing, and recording data	2—Assessing data	3—Managing problems and maintaining health
A Attitudes	A1 Continually monitors patients' conditions and records essential data in legible fashion. Assesses pre-illness feelings of parents toward child. Avoids stereotyped data gathering behavior which would unduly delay other tasks.	A2 Faced with unfamiliar fluid and electrolyte problem, calls consultant promptly.	A3 Interested and available to answer family's questions about prognosis. Record reflects adequate plan for follow up care.
B Factual knowledge	B1 States major and minor signs and symptoms of meningitis correctly.	B2 States principal causes of meningitis and complications correctly.	B3 States minimal length of treatment correctly. Explains why inappropriate ADH secretions may complicate treatment and what the signs might be.
C Interpersonal skills	C1 Accepts the sometimes inappropriate attitudes of the family of a seriously ill child, yet still communicates feelings of concern, urgency, and reassurance so as to obtain reliable data.	C2 Explains working diagnosis to family in appropriate manner.	C3 Explains treatment plan to family at their level of comprehension. Is able to obtain informed consent comfortably. Avoids condescension in answering trivial questions.
D Technical skills	D1 Skillfully carries out lumbar puncture, spinal fluid cell count, and stained smear for organism identification.	D2 Can recognize gram negative pleomorphic organism on Gram stain.	D3 Correctly starts and maintains I.V. Gives intramuscular or subcutaneous injection safely.
E Clinical judgment	E1 Is appropriately persistent in efforts to obtain cerebrospinal fluid sample and blood culture. Realizes when to turn from data gathering to other tasks.	E2 Displays logic in interpretation of data as obtained and with data complete can state the problem clearly.	E3 Implements appropriate action. Recognizes and deals appropriately with the complications most likely to develop, including iatrogenic ones or nosocomial accidents. Is able to revise diagnostic hypotheses on basis of new data.

American Board of Pediatrics, Inc. 1974. Foundations for Evaluating the Competency of Pediatrics. Chicago: American Board of Pediatrics, Inc. Reprinted by permission.

THE DIMENSIONS OF FUNCTIONAL
DOMAIN AND DYSFUNCTION: CONTENT

The development of the matrix has not fully answered the original concern of the Board that it needed a way of relating the *content* of its examination to the *competencies* required of pediatricians. In years past, the Board has used familiar and traditional content categories to catalog the examination material in terms of organ systems, etiologic factors, ages of patients, locus of encounter (office versus emergency room versus hospital), and others (for example, care of illness versus health maintenance versus prevention). A recent analysis of one of the Board's examinations suggested that it might be more fruitful to redefine the content categories of the examination, with the specification of two new dimensions: *functional domain* (analogous to organ system), and *dysfunction* (reflecting etiology). The initial choice of functional domains and of dysfunctions is indicated in Figure 3. The functional domains include such categories as psychology and behavior, body fluids, intermediary metabolism, and multiple systems, along with other more traditional designations of organ systems. Dysfunctions include the categories of developmental and psychophysiologic, metabolic (either genetic or acquired), nutritional, toxic, traumatic, idiopathic, and iatrogenic. A review of a recent examination of the ABP indicated that a small number of test questions, easily classified with respect to functional domain, demanded only a statement about diagnostic procedure, therapeutic method, or some identifying basic science characteristic to be classified along the second dimension; accordingly, these three categories of interaction with functional domains were added to the matrix.

When the questions on the examination were assigned to the various cells of the matrix as logically as possible, albeit somewhat arbitrarily, the surprising discovery was made that there was only one question that dealt with infectious problems involving the ear, nose, throat, or larynx, out of a total of nearly 200 questions. Another question dealt with infections of the lower respiratory tract. This analysis begs the question as to whether there were only two aspects of care of infectious problems of the respiratory tract that deserved questions, problems in this area being among those most commonly seen by pediatricians. The selection of two content items in this area would never be acceptable from the standpoint of education, since the goal of the educator is to identify for the student all the relevant content within *each cell* of the matrix. The goal of the evaluator, on the other hand, is to see that the cells of the *matrix as a whole* are *sampled* in such as way as to give a reliable estimate of the overall competency. There is no reason to assume that the dimensions or the content of the sample should exactly match the activities of the physician, especially in

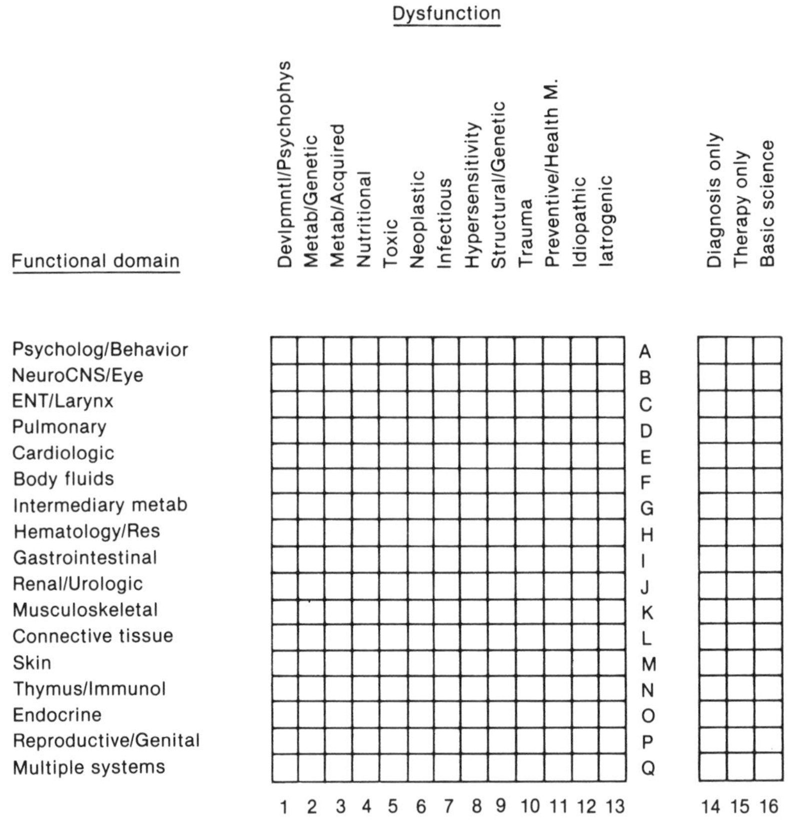

Dysfunction

Functional domain — column headers (vertical):
Devlpmnt/Psychophys, Metab/Genetic, Metab/Acquired, Nutritional, Toxic, Neoplastic, Infectious, Hypersensitivity, Structural/Genetic, Trauma, Preventive/Health M., Idiopathic, Iatrogenic, Diagnosis only, Therapy only, Basic science

Functional domain		Row
Psycholog/Behavior		A
NeuroCNS/Eye		B
ENT/Larynx		C
Pulmonary		D
Cardiologic		E
Body fluids		F
Intermediary metab		G
Hematology/Res		H
Gastrointestinal		I
Renal/Urologic		J
Musculoskeletal		K
Connective tissue		L
Skin		M
Thymus/Immunol		N
Endocrine		O
Reproductive/Genital		P
Multiple systems		Q

1 2 3 4 5 6 7 8 9 10 11 12 13   14 15 16

Figure 3.   Content matrix with the dimensions of functional domain and dysfunction.

noncritical or trivial areas; but the use of the matrix may help this sampling process become more optimally rational and valid.

In any case, if the content relevant to any cell or group of cells in the matrix were so crucial to the competency of pediatricians that an examination must reliably test and certify to competence in those cells alone, then there should be a large enough number of questions dealing with the content of those cells to permit reliable judgments to be made. An implication of this might be that examinations would become longer in order to provide reliable samples in all crucial areas identified.

The notions of functional domain and dysfunction have been referred to as dimensions, but they are not truly scalar; rather, they represent a set of *structures* on the one hand, and *processes* on the other. There are other aspects of pediatric practice that have more truly or nearly scalar aspects. For example, a concern with problems of certain age groups would generate the categories of fetus/newborn, child, or adolescent; the continuum of clinical care might generate prevention, screening, diagnosis, treatment, follow-up, and health maintenance; a concern with the level of intensity of care might identify office or outpatient clinic, institutions for chronic care, emergency room, or hospital wards, nurseries or intensive care units; and an interest in the role of the physician might identify problems belonging to primary care, to consultant activities or academic or administrative roles, or to tertiary care.

We believe that it has been helpful to set the nonscalar categories of functional domains and dysfunctions (identifying structures and processes) apart from these other dimensions. It is entirely possible, though, for a computer to store examination questions identified with respect to all of these characteristics, to enumerate the characteristics on demand, and to recall any or all questions having specified characteristics. As we have manipulated these matrices, it has become apparent that the *content matrix is very helpful in developing and cataloging the material appropriate for education or for evaluation*, and that the *competency* matrix helps us to know how to develop a given item of content in terms of the skills and tasks needed to deal with it. When both the educational program and the evaluation program address the same identified set of competencies, the goals of both programs can be made congruent and comprehensive.

APPLICATION TO DEVELOPMENTAL DISABILITIES

Another opportunity to examine the application of a content matrix came with the work of the Subcommittee on Curriculum in Normal Human Development and Developmental Disabilities of the American Association of University Affiliated Programs, which has twice met to try to define the curriculum appropriate in medicine for those who will be responsible for patients with developmental disabilities. The content matrix was introduced, however, only after a discussion of the general competency matrix.

At its first meeting, the Subcommittee examined the proposition that it might be more productive in the long run to specify the goals, rather than the content, of education for care of children with developmental disabilities and their families, especially if this can be done in such terms that progress toward achievement of these goals can be reliably and validly evaluated (See Chapter 16, this volume, for an amplification of this point.) For each of the 15 cells of the matrix in Figure 1, general statements can be made about the kind of physician who can effectively care for the developmentally disabled. For example, cell A-2 lodges attitudes toward assessment. We would want a physician to be: 1) tolerant of uncertainty, rather than making premature judgments regarding the patients seen; 2) able to use uncertainty to mobilize further information; 3) able to redirect inquiry, change the direction of study, or acknowledge the need to change a diagnosis when appropriate; or 4) able to give evidence of a nonjudgmental acceptance of nonconformity and human variability. These attributes of attitude will be, on the whole, very difficult to assess in any way except through supervision of the practice of physicians in training and through knowledge of how they function in the actual clinical setting.

The potential for evaluation is quite different when we study a cell like B-2 (Figure 1), which asks for cognitive skills with respect to the task of assessment. It will be possible to name a host of items that we feel physicians responsible for the care of children with developmental disabilities and their families should know about the assessment of historical, clinical, and laboratory data. The depth of knowledge will vary with the level of education of the student or practitioner, or with the levels of responsibility assumed, but the knowledge required can be often stated with a high degree of precision, as an aid to both education and evaluation. For example, we might ask the physician in a second year of pediatric residency to be able to recognize the following syndromes from photographs of typically affected children: Down's syndrome, hypothyroid infant, trisomy 18, spastic diplegia, microcephaly, 2 out of 3 craniosynotoses (Crouzon, Apert, or scaphocephaly), cherry red spot, gingival hypertrophy (phenytoin), achondroplasia, Treacher Collins syndrome, ataxia-telangiectasis, Cornelia de Lange syndrome, or·mucopolysaccharidoses. We might ask the same physician to recognize petit mal, myoclonic seizures, rheumatic chorea in typical motion picture films or television tapes. Or we could ask that he/she present a reasonable differential diagnosis between tuberculous meningitis, Guillain-Barré syndrome, lead intoxication, suppressed pyogenic meningitis, acute viral meningoencephalitis, and brain abscess, on the basis of likely clinical signs, cerebrospinal fluid findings and other appropriate laboratory studies, with the indications for such other studies.

When educational goals are stated with such precision, when they are shared with the student, and when the student knows that a coherent evaluation procedure congruent with the stated goals is proposed, then the student has the best chance of being able to develop those abilities and skills that will make him/her competent to accomplish the tasks presented by clinical problems. An intelligent curriculum will follow, making appropriate uses of the student's point of departure, of his/her learning style, of the knowledge and supervisory skills of teachers, and of the local clinical research, and educational resources.

Function, dysfunction, task, basic science

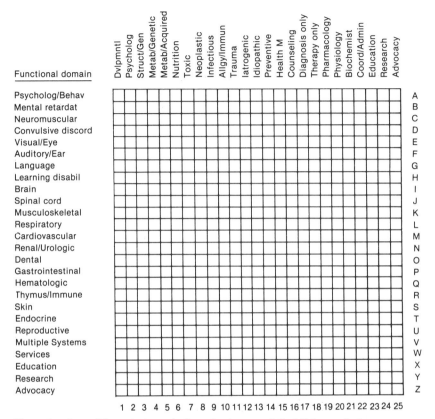

Figure 4. A possible content matrix for a developmental disabilities curriculum.

In the further development of curriculum for developmental disabilities, the competency matrix can be usefully complemented by a content matrix. Figure 4 indicates a tentative form for such a matrix. The importance of convulsive disorders, language disabilities, or learning disabilities to the general field of developmental disabilities seems to warrant the exposure of each as a functional domain. The process coordinate might separate developmental and psychologic disabilities, as well as contain counseling, coordination/administration, education, research, and advocacy, in addition to processes relevant to general pediatrics (see Figure 4). Services, education, research, and advocacy may also appear as functional domains, where they would have somewhat different meanings. This matrix contains 650 cells! And it may still be incomplete!

A matrix of 650 cells may be grossly redundant or hypertrophied. On the other hand, it represents an arbitrary choice of items, some of which may be more useful than others. In a large matrix many of the cells may be meaningless or empty; others will have trivial content; and others will be important for some purposes, but not for others. For example, cell W-22 (Figure 4), which deals with the coordination and administration of services to the developmentally disabled, may be relatively irrelevant for medical students, whereas it would have high priority in both the training and the evaluation of those preparing for responsible positions in direction of academic or service programs.

For any content matrix to become maximally useful, it should be developed by those who will use it, with reasonable agreement as to how functional domains and processes are to be defined and where the assignment is to be made of content items for which the assignment is not clear or is possible in two or more ways. Categories in either the structural or the process areas can be consolidated or expanded in accordance with need while other categories are eliminated or added.

The competency matrix has already been used extensively by the Examination Committees of the American Board of Pediatrics (ABP) and by the Task Forces of the Joint Committee on Recertification of the American Board of Pediatrics and the American Academy of Pediatrics in the development of certifying and recertifying examinations. A content matrix will be used in indexing the examinations of the ABP and in developing the feedback to be given candidates, which will indicate to them the content of questions for which incorrect answers were given. The purpose of this feedback is to identify areas of incomplete knowledge, as a guide to self-evaluation and appropriate remedial continuing education.

I suggest that as we look at the problem of education of physicians for the care of persons with developmental disabilities, we may find it helpful to organize our thoughts about curriculum and about evaluation around the notions, both implicit and explicit, which are embodied in competency and content matrices such as these.

ACKNOWLEDGMENT

I should like to thank the American Board of Pediatrics for the privilege of sharing information regarding its examinations.

REFERENCES

American Board of Pediatrics, Inc. 1974. Foundations for Evaluating the Competency of Pediatricians. Chicago: American Board of Pediatrics, Inc.
Burg, F. D., Brownlee, R. C., Wright, F. H., Levine, H., Daeschner, C. W., Vaughan, V. C., III, and Anderson, J. A. 1976. A method for defining competency in pediatrics. Journal of Medical Education, 51, 824–828.

chapter 7

CURRICULUM IN HANDICAPPING CONDITIONS
Implications for Residency, Fellowship, and Continuing Education of Pediatricians

Donald W. Delaney, John B. Bartram, Richard W. Olmsted, and Stephen C. Copps

Pediatric education in the future must provide residents and practicing pediatricians with the skills to evaluate and support the development of all children — nonhandicapped and handicapped alike. Today, approximately one-third of the pediatric residencies have no teaching program that focuses on the needs of exceptional children and their families. In the many that do provide such programs, the experience is often unstructured or elective. Yet recent trends in pediatric practice coupled with recent social/educational legislation (most importantly, perhaps, Public Law 94-142) have brought an increasing emphasis on child development and handicapping conditions in residency programs. In addition, fellowship opportunities in these fields have proliferated and new interest in continuing education efforts has developed along related lines. The purpose of this chapter is to consider the implications of such curricular changes at the residency, fellowship, and continuing education levels.

RESIDENCY TRAINING

Although a comprehensive residency program in this area can take many forms with a wide range of goals and objectives (see Chapter 16, this volume, for a summary), this section of the chapter discusses and analyzes six key educational objectives.

Educational Objective 1: To understand and utilize a fund of knowledge of developmental pediatrics. It is a challenge to the training program director to construct a vigorous, demanding, and rewarding curriculum that enables the residents to not only progressively accumulate knowledge of development and developmental abnormalities, but also convinces them that this is an important and exciting area. Within the hospital setting the faculty and residents are distracted from this area by the more acute care needs of the child. Rapidly changing pathophysiology and the immediate gratification that results from the feeling that one is taking part in the interruption of these pathologic processes is tough competition indeed. But this competition for time and effort need not exist. Even though the child is present within the acute care setting for a very short segment of his/her developing years, the child can teach us a great deal about development if we do not concentrate on the disease process alone, but on the developing child as well.

An additional challenge is that the subject matter of developmental pediatrics is vast and diffuse. Developmentalists themselves will define developmental pediatrics in different ways. Some stress the basic science of normal development, some focus on behavior, and others emphasize mental retardation or neurologic developmental problems. As a result, each developmentalist has a bias when advising a curriculum committee.

Nevertheless, there is a body of didactic knowledge of child development that can be presented in the conference room and through demonstrations in the playroom and in the child's classroom. But the application of this knowledge must also take place through reinforcement and repetition in more typical settings, such as the sick child's bedside or the clinic setting. It is our contention that this can only be successfully carried out by model pediatricians who have a deep commitment and love of teaching around the developing child.

Educational Objective 2: To demonstrate an accepting attitude toward the exceptional child and his/her altered lifestyle. A society that prides itself on the intellectual achievements of its members to the extent that our society does creates a competitiveness for accomplishment and a devaluation of the child who can compete less well than his/her peers. It is within memory that plans for institutionalization of children born with Down's syndrome were started at the time of birth. Sometimes the physician displays a feeling of resignation of effort, a suggestion of indifference, or a subtle disrespect for the resultant lifestyle of the more severely affected child. Perceptive parents sense this, and, although not able to articulate their feelings, may respond with hostility or noncompliance, or they may set expectations for the child that fall short of the child's potential. Since society has not yet developed a more accepting attitude for such children, residents need a program of "debriefing" or "de-learning" of this attitude early on in their training program.

Educational Objective 3: To be an effective member of a team of health professionals. The development of the pediatrician as an effective team member starts with the expectations of the training program director that the PL-1 will develop both self-respect and respect for others competent in their helping roles within the program. This feeling of mutual respect is the foundation for the development of good professional relationships and an esprit de corps. This must permeate the whole program before a team of professionals caring for the exceptional child and his/her family can successfully accomplish its goals. The definition of roles of all members of the team must be clear, mutually understood, and communicated to the family and, when appropriate, the child.

The pediatrician, when responsible for the primary care of the child, will usually assume the role of coordinator of the team. Coordination means harmonious adjustment or functioning, a task that calls for time, energy, and diplomacy, from which immediate gratification may be lacking. Coordination calls for an understanding of the language and the concepts of the various disciplines and also requires the ability to translate these concepts into functional terms understandable by parents and teachers. On the other hand, the pediatrician's role may become a consultative one, especially as the educational needs of the child are planned. Again, he/she must recognize, and then utilize in the health plan, the skills and contributions of these experts. The pediatrician must remain involved in an advocacy role raising constructive questions for the benefit of the child and his/her family.

The role of medicine in carrying out Public Law 94-142 has not been adequately defined and will vary between jurisdictions (see Palfrey, Mervis, and Butler, 1978), but it is probable that parents, educators, and school district officials will turn to medicine for help in the identification and program planning of exceptional children. It is important that the pediatrician realize the limitations inherent in the tools now available in order to assist the health care team to make realistic projections.

Educational Objective 4: To counsel families regarding development of the handicapped child. Nurturing the child to maximize development to his/her potential with the least amount of physical, emotional, and intellectual trauma calls for an accepting atmosphere in the home, free of guilt, self-blame, or the blaming of others. Parental and sibling anxiety must be recognized and understood, especially during the time that family members are learning to alter and then accept their revised expectations for the exceptional child (see Chapter 4, this volume). The parents, as nurturers of the child, need the nurturing of the empathetic pediatrician. The pediatrician may need to provide anticipatory empathetic guidance, as well as being a stable, consistent, and dependable force in what seems to be a chaotic world. If this quality can be taught at all, it may best be accomplished by the utilization of a role model in the training program.

Educational Objective 5: To develop and utilize knowledge of pharmacological agents. Resident instruction must include information about the relatively new and expanding pharmacological agents used in organically and psychologically based behavior disorders. The application of these agents must be more than casual prescription writing. Graduating residents should be aware of the side effects and the combined effects of two or more drugs. They also must be aware of the pressure applied from parents, teachers, and counselors to use these agents. Finally, the resident should be aware of the ethical and moral issues surrounding the use of children in clinical drug studies and of the adverse feelings of some regarding drug alteration of a child's behavior.

Educational Objective 6: To understand the principles of research. A basic understanding of research methodology and the ability to incorporate this methodology in daily patient care should be an essential part of the training program. Moreover, the development of better tools for evaluating the child, for evaluating the effectiveness of interaction strategies, and for developing more effective means of enhancing the development of handicapped children should also be included in the training program. The involvement of community pediatricians in research and evaluation programs is something that should be more prevalent. For example, the pediatrician is often in the best position to discover those factors that cause some families to grow with adversity while others buckle under.

Barriers to Curriculum Development

With these goals as background, it is important now to identify the many difficulties that face the training director of a residency program in developing and implementing a curriculum incorporating these educational objectives. First, the medical model, evolving over hundreds of years, has become the basis for clinical medical education and has served us well. However, the model is a clinical entity and disease-oriented one, which is not a useful model for many aspects of a handicapped child curriculum. We have all been part of or witnessed the anxiety produced in a medical team by a child for whom we cannot place a label. Often by that very labeling we may be limiting a child through a "tracking system" and may be discouraging caretakers from setting realistic, often higher, expectations. Certainly the medical model should not be dispensed with, but when dealing with the exceptional child a more functional model that includes an identification of the child's capabilities should be utilized. Acceptance of the relevance of different models is an important but difficult step.

Second, in this day of cost accounting, cost effectiveness, and cost control we are examining closely the price of resident education. House staff stipends must be justified to third party payers. Time spent involved in educational activities by house staff is coming under close scrutiny and may not be paid for in the traditional fashion in the future. The curriculum for teaching about exceptional children who are not in the acute care setting may need to be paid for in some other way. Clearly, this is a potentially major barrier to curriculum implementation in this area.

Finally, the amount of time that we allocate for this aspect of our residency program has not been defined. If we accept the figure that 10%-12% of the children can be categorized as exceptional and if we can apportion training time in accordance with incidence figures, then obviously we need to drastically change our present allocation of time in residency training. Should the time spent in this area be in proportion to the incidence of handicapping conditions within the population? We have not used this formula in other areas. Rather, we have been pressured to meet the acute service needs of the institution and have weighted the programs too heavily in some areas, such as neonatology, and too lightly in other areas, such as developmental pediatrics and the exceptional child. Thus, the present time allocation poses another significant but not insurmountable barrier.

FELLOWSHIP TRAINING

A focus on the development of fellowship curricula for programs to educate and train pediatric specialists to work more effectively with exceptional children is based upon a number of premises and facts. First, there is a significantly large number of children who require special long-term care as a result of organically and/or environmentally based problems, which lead to prolonged difficulty in learning, problems in self-concept, deficits in physical and social functioning, and difficulties in adapting to the expectations of parents and others. Second, there are several professions, including pediatrics, that are or should be concerned with the provision of this special type of care. The average pediatrician or family doctor cannot look forward to providing this care adequately without help from others. Third, changes in conventional pediatric training programs are essential if pediatrics is to provide leadership and make a significant contribution to the care of the developmentally disabled.

A number of groups around the country have independently come to conclusions as to the basic content of a fellowship program for pediatricians (see Chapter 12, this volume). In addition to at least 2 years of general pediatric residency (and in many cases a few years in general pediatric practice as well), there seems to be agreement that fellows should have or should acquire special skills and aptitudes in the following areas:

1. Child development, with an appreciation of the organic and environmental factors that affect children both positively and negatively.
2. Genetic disorders and counseling, metabolic diseases, sensory deficits, and the value of total communication, pediatric neurology (particularly the management of seizures and CNS defects), learning, emotional problems of children, and legal issues.
3. A comfortable, workable understanding of parent/child relationships, particularly during early infancy, and of the parent/professional and parent/child discords that are common to those in daily contact with the handicapped.
4. Positive attitudes and understanding in relation to communicating with family, child, and other professionals, especially those from the areas of education, social work, psychology, and language development.
5. Administrative skills and working knowledge of governmental procedures, public health operations, and community resources.

These last few content areas appear to be best acquired in an ongoing service setting where good role models are available. Fellowship programs should endeavor to teach the art of month-to-month and year-to-year management, as well as provide opportunities for fellows to make differential diagnoses or to engage in emergency care. In addition to providing expert medical management, the fellow should accept the responsibility of providing support to children and families, whether nuclear, single parent, or extended, in solving nonmedical problems. The fellow should also become aware of and be involved in ethical, social, economic, and political dilemmas associated with the care of the exceptional child.

Certification in Developmental Pediatrics and Fellowship Curricula

All pediatricians should have competency not only in the area of applied child development but also in the management of children who, for a variety of reasons, have long-term problems in which cure is not anticipated. Nevertheless, it appears that specialization leading to certification in this area is essential. The general pediatrician will rarely take the necessary time to spend with children and their families, nor does he/she have ample knowledge of community resources to make appropriate use of other individuals and organizations. A relatively small group of pediatric specialists in practice, teaching centers, or interdisciplinary community programs is essential to provide high quality care. Certification as a pediatric subspecialty is necessary in order to establish minimal standards of skills and knowledge and to provide recognition and appropriate reimbursement for this special service. Moreover, all physicians need increased competence in this area, and teaching responsibilities at the internship and residency level for pediatricians and family practitioners should fall to such specialists.

As a result of the efforts of Arnold Capute and Lawrence Taft, the American Board of Pediatrics has initiated action to establish certification for pediatric specialists in the area of developmental disabilities. Hopefully, as these plans develop, there will be better integration of the efforts among those concerned primarily with developmental pediatrics and pediatric habilitation and those from the fields of physical medicine and rehabilitation, and pediatric neurology. It would seem appropriate for these groups and for chairpersons of pediatric departments to develop jointly the goals of training and the basic content of programs and curricula leading to high standards of competency in the care of the exceptional child, as well as to attempt to measure the effectiveness of such programs.

Concern currently expressed by the University Affiliated Programs, the Bureau of Community Health Services, State Departments of Health, State Developmental Disabilities Councils, the White House Conference on Handicapped Individuals, the National Board of Medical Examiners, the Section on Child Development and the Committee on the Handicapped Child of the American Academy of Pediatrics, the Bureau of Education for the Handicapped, parent and voluntary health organizations, as well as other professional groups relating to the handicapped, attests to the general interest in better professional training in developmental pediatrics and the need for such specialists.

CONTINUING EDUCATION

In planning teaching programs at the continuing education level regarding exceptional children, it is helpful to know certain trends that are occurring in pediatric practice and in the educational needs of pediatricians. The recent Manpower Survey conducted by the American Academy of Pediatrics and by the Task Force on Pediatric Education (1978) indicates that pediatricians are being called upon, with increasing frequency, to provide services for children and adolescents with problems of a behavioral, emotional, and educational nature. A survey of mothers' opinions regarding health care of their children indicated that many of them would utilize the resources of a pediatrician for problems of a biosocial nature if they realized that pediatricians were interested in these problems. The majority of mothers also said they would be willing to pay for such services if they were available.

In addition to survey data, the Task Force on Pediatric Education has documented the changing nature of the health needs of children and adolescents. It is clear that these health needs are increasing in the biosocial and educational realm. Accordingly, the Task Force has recommended that there be much more attention given to the teaching of biosocial pediatrics, particularly at the resident level. A further recommendation of the Task Force is the need for special emphasis on teaching relative to the care of the child with multiple handicaps and chronic illness.

A large number of pediatricians practicing general pediatrics indicate that they have an area of special interest; an even larger number indicate that they would like to develop such an interest. Competence in an area of special interest may be gained through an additional year or more of residency training or through continuing education efforts and on-the-job training. It is significant that aside from allergy, the areas of special interest most preferred are in the biosocial and educational spheres. Pediatric departments and training programs may find great demand from pediatricians with interests in developmental disabilities to have continuing education programs in this specific area. Continuing education efforts may take the form of participation by the pediatrician in specialty clinics and other clinical settings in addition to didactic teaching.

Perhaps the most exciting recent developments are the Pediatrics Review and Education Program (1978) of the American Academy of Pediatrics and the Program for Continuing Education and Assessment Leading to Recertification in Pediatrics (1978) of the American Board of Pediatrics. For the first time, educational objectives, a curriculum, and an evaluation process will be coordinated for continuing education available to all pediatricians. In addition to a review of recent advances in pediatrics, during each year of a 6-year program, special topics for review will be offered. Among the topics for annual review are growth and development, behavioral pediatrics, mental retardation, genetics and dysmorphism, learning disabilities and school adjustment problems, and the handicapped child. Examination for recertification by the American Board of Pediatrics will cover the same topics as the Academy's Pediatrics Review and Education Program. Consequently, it appears that the needs and interests of practicing pediatricians to gain a greater knowledge in the area of developmental pediatrics can be accomplished through such continuing education efforts.

CONCLUSIONS

This overview of a curriculum in handicapping conditions for various training levels suggests a clear need for such a curriculum as well as possible content, educational strategies, and the barriers to implementation.

Despite the fact that the training needs of practicing pediatricians, fellows, and residents are quite different, there exists a pool of knowledge, skills, and attitudes shared by all levels. It is recommended that a comprehensive educational approach identify both the common and differing goals of a curriculum related to exceptional children.

REFERENCES

Palfrey, J. D., Mervis, R. C., and Butler, J. A. 1978. New directions in the evaluation and education of handicapped children. New England Journal of Medicine, 298, 819–824.
Pediatric Review and Education Program. 1978. Evanston, Ill.: American Academy of Pediatrics.
Program for Continuing Education and Assessment Leading to Recertification in Pediatrics. 1978. Chapel Hill, N.C.: American Board of Pediatrics.
The Task Force on Pediatric Education. 1978. The Future of Pediatric Education. Evanston, Ill.: American Academy of Pediatrics.

IMPLEMENTATION AND EVALUATION OF PROGRAMS

chapter 8

A MEDICAL STUDENT CURRICULUM ON THE NEEDS OF EXCEPTIONAL CHILDREN

Marvin I. Gottlieb and Peter W. Zinkus

The presumed uniqueness of the exceptional child is fashioned by an amalgamation of several interdependent factors: 1) the relatively complex nature of the primary disability, 2) the occurrence of multiple secondary disturbances, 3) the protracted, often life-long, course of the disorder, and 4) the pervasive complications of the problem, which often extend beyond the family constellation to involve the community. As a rule, exceptionality implies a chronic disorder that influences various facets of physical, social, psychological, and educational development. Unfortunately the categorization as *exceptional* almost automatically evokes feelings of hopelessness and despair for the patient and the family. Frequently this aura of pessimism is exaggerated as a result of professional anxiety, which may be engendered by inadequate training and, therefore, a lack of enthusiasm. Perhaps the labeling of the child as exceptional is, in part, the professional's admission of an inability to cope with chronic handicapping conditions of childhood. The quality of a teaching curriculum that focuses on the needs of the exceptional child is significant in that it may directly influence the attitudes of medical students and the nature of their subsequent professional intervention.

The Section of Developmental and Behavioral Pediatrics, The University of Tennessee Center for the Health Sciences/Le Bonheur Children's Hospital (UTCHS/LBCH) is dedicated to providing a quality teaching curriculum and to developing positive professional attitudes with regard to the care and treatment of handicapped children and their families. *All* medical students at the UTCHS/LBCH are introduced to the diverse ramifications of chronic handicapping disorders of childhood through several educational modalities, including: didactic presentations, clinical experiences, conference groups, and self-study programs. A medically oriented interdisciplinary faculty participates in the teaching program, presenting a spectrum of exceptional problems: developmental delays, learning disabilities, mental retardation, neurologic handicaps, behavioral disorders, and emotional disturbances. The teaching model attempts to encourage a holistic perspective of patient, family, and community as they are affected by disorders of this type. The educational philosophy stresses that the keys to dissipating the paralyzing myths about exceptionality are: 1) a broad familiarity with the various entities comprising chronic handicapping disorders, 2) a recognition of the need for medical intervention with exceptional children, 3) an appreciation of the profound consequences of these disorders on patient and family, 4) an awareness of available and needed community resources, and 5) an ability to effectively cooperate with an interdisciplinary team.

**DEVELOPMENT AND
ADMINISTRATIVE STRUCTURE OF THE PROGRAM**

In early 1970, the Department of Pediatrics formally introduced a service-teaching-research module in developmental and behavioral pediatrics as part of the pediatric core curriculum for medical students. The program was incorporated into the Ambulatory Pediatric Service teaching module; a mandatory rotation for the 200 medical students (annually) enrolled in the University of Tennessee Center for the Health Sciences. The *Clinic for Exceptional Children* was established as a specialty service to provide clinical experiences in developmental and behavioral disabilities for the students. The Department of Pediatrics encouraged the expansion of the teaching model, and in 1977 it was formally organized as a *Section of Developmental and Behavioral Pediatrics* to supervise the training program for medical students, interns, and pediatric residents.

Each year the program has been modified to expand the scope of teaching in exceptionality and to accommodate the increasing number of elective students. The faculty of the Section has been increased to more effectively cover the spectrum of exceptional problems. Full-time faculty includes a pediatrician, a services coordinator, a clinical psychologist, a pediatric nurse practitioner, a psychometrist, social workers, a speech/language therapist, and a special educator. In addition, several part-time faculty participate in clinic activities: an audiologist, a child development specialist, an ophthalmology resident, an otolaryngology resident, a pedodontia resident, a social work graduate student, and speech/language graduate students.

The Section functions within the traditional organizational format of the University and receives administrative support as part of the University structure. In essence, the teaching of exceptional problems has become a very structured and integral component of the UTCHS/LBCH pediatric training program.

GOALS, OBJECTIVES, AND OVERVIEW

The broad teaching responsibilities of the Section of Developmental and Behavioral Pediatrics focuses on various aspects of the exceptional child and his/her family. Some of the broad goals of the teaching program for medical students include:

1. To expand and enhance the pediatric training of medical students by including problems of exceptionality in the core curriculum.
2. To present problems of the exceptional child in the context of an ambulatory pediatric service, thereby de-emphasizing the uniqueness of the exceptional child and encouraging the recognition of these problems as an integral part of comprehensive health care.
3. To augment the medical student's fund of basic medical knowledge by presenting problems in identification and therapeutic management of exceptional children through clinical and didactic experiences.
4. To encourage medical students to approach exceptional problems in a realistic, active, and confident manner. This is accomplished in part by simulating a private practice setting; offering office management, demonstrating methods of securing additional professional diagnostic assistance, and having students become familiar with community resources.
5. To support the concept of a medically oriented interdisciplinary approach to comprehensive health care services by including medical students in the "team" effort. This model provides opportunities for direct student contact with social workers, speech pathologists, psychologists, special educators, and others.

One of our major concerns is with the child from early infancy to school age. Disturbances in development and behavior observed in the older child are frequently a reflection of problems encountered during infancy and early childhood. Attention is therefore focused on early detection of potential disabilities, family relationships, attitudes, and early medical intervention. The program for medical students also emphasizes the issues of prevention of exceptionality as well as detection and therapy.

Experiences for the medical student that stress early childhood development include participation in: periodic developmental screening of infants and children, group programs for parents, workshops for community facilities (e.g., day care centers), and programs for foster care providers. Additional experiences include observation of preschool training programs for children with developmental delays, the development of home learning materials for stimulating and enhancing child development, as well as consultation with preschool programs.

TEACHING MODULE UTILIZED FOR MEDICAL STUDENT ROTATION

With regard to clinical experiences, two student teaching models have been designed. The *private practice-oriented model* (Figure 1) was designed to simulate experiences as encountered in either a pediatric or family practice office setting. The student evaluates the child with a suspected developmental or behavioral prcblem, utilizing his/her own medical resources and expertise while being assisted by a pediatric nurse associate. The medical evaluation includes a comprehensive history (obtained from the parents), a teacher contact, physical and neurological examinations, and a developmental screening. After completing the examination, the student meets with the clinic director and selected staff to review the findings. Discussion focuses on observations made during the evaluation, the differential diagnosis suggested, additional intervention needed to clarify or define the diagnosis, professionals to be consulted (e.g., psychologist), and the approximate cost of the evaluation. In addition, the conference reviews the coordination of an interdisciplinary effort, the parent informing-interview, and the follow-up services required. The private-practice model is a reality-based approach to exceptional children. A perspective of "what I could do if I were out in the world of practice" is simulated.

The *academically-oriented model* (Figure 2) provides a more in-depth clinical experience for the medical student. During this clinic session, the patient and his/her family are evaluated by an interdisciplinary team (medical students, a social worker, a speech pathologist, an audiologist, a pediatric nurse associate, a special educator, and other selected professionals).

The medical students become an integral and active part of this interdisciplinary interaction. During the conference, the team findings are reviewed, coordinated, and summarized for reports. The need for further investigation, the differential diagnosis, and the therapeutic recommendations are analyzed and projected. The students are part of this process and incorporate their findings into the framework of a holistic diagnostic screening. They are encouraged to question findings of other team members and to explore results of specific test findings reported by other pro-

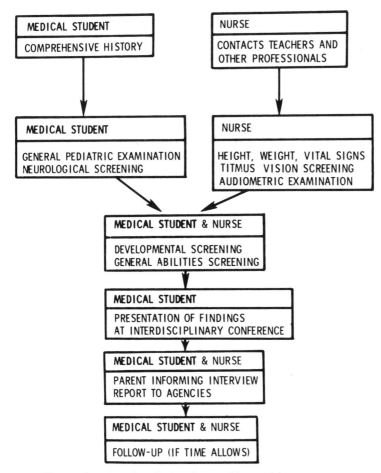

Figure 1. The practice-oriented medical student teaching model

fessionals. In addition, students are urged to participate in follow-up services. Records are kept within the clinic facility allowing students to periodically check the progress of their patients.

In addition to clinical experiences, associated staff conferences, and informal discussions, several didactic approaches to the exceptional child are utilized. This includes a series of lectures, television tape reviews, and slide presentations on issues relating to exceptional problems in developmental and behavioral pediatrics. In addition, a self-study program is available in the clinic library, which includes a series of television tapes, programmed audio-visual lectures, audiotapes, and texts on issues related to exceptional children. A variety of discussions are conducted informally to assist students in their appreciation of the program, the problems encountered, and their specific roles in medicine.

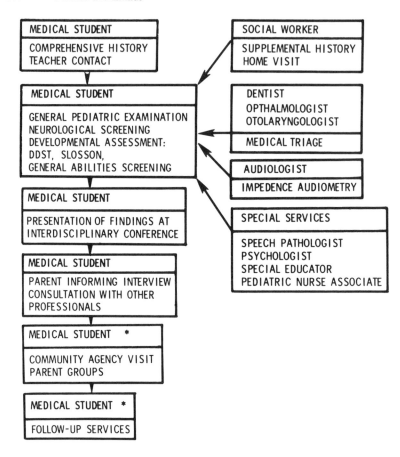

Figure 2.   The academically-oriented medical student teaching model

TEACHING MODULE UTILIZED FOR MEDICAL STUDENT ELECTIVE

In addition to the curriculum previously reviewed for medical students in
pediatrics, an elective program is offered. The elective is a block rotation
and allows for an expanded training model for medical students. The elective program incorporates additional teaching experiences, such as: 1) patient follow-up — providing opportunities for supervised continuum
care; 2) field trip experiences — including visits, supervised by members
of the interdisciplinary faculty, to a variety of community resources serving exceptional children; 3) counseling — providing students with opportunities to participate in individual family and group counseling sessions;
4) teaching — in which medical students act in a supervisory capacity at
various clinic sessions, assisting in the teaching of graduate students from

the various disciplines assigned to the clinic; and 5) research — in which interested students participate in ongoing research programs.

Finally, as part of the elective program, medical students meet individually with members of the interdisciplinary faculty. Time is allocated for in-depth staff meetings with individual faculty members and with groups. Pertinent reading materials are assigned and discussed. Informal discussions are periodically arranged to review the student's needs and goals in medicine as they relate to the exceptional child.

SUMMARY

As this training program has evolved, we have identified a number of critical concepts that are summarized below. As noted, the program's philosophy emphasizes the holistic approach to child care. Opportunities are provided for screening of developmental and behavioral problems within the ambulatory pediatric experience, with additional opportunities for a more comprehensive evaluation of the patient. Developmental and behavioral pediatrics is incorporated in the general training of physicians, thereby de-emphasizing the exceptional nature of these problems. In addition, the program is designed to introduce medical students and students of allied health professions to the interdisciplinary approach to comprehensive health care services early in their training. The interdisciplinary team is medically oriented, and one of its goals is medical student teaching. Student interaction with the interdisciplinary professional team fosters better understanding and communication among health care specialists. Teaching and service are amalgamated into a meaningful program, one augmenting the other. Students with either practice or academic career orientations have opportunities for varying levels of study of developmental and behavioral problems. They are provided with opportunities not only to identify problems but to become familiar with community resources for therapeutic intervention. Accordingly, the Section and Clinic serve as a nucleus for developing cohesiveness between a variety of community agencies.

Medical students are indoctrinated into a new philosophy of pediatric medicine, a philosophy which stresses a child's development in its broadest context. The pediatric health care team is challenged with providing diagnostic and therapeutic intervention for children with a myriad of exceptional problems: developmental lags, learning disabilities, communication disorders, perceptual disturbances, intellectual deficits, behavioral and emotional problems. A critical challenge is to help the medical student develop enthusiasm for this phase of child care and to think in terms of early detection and meaningful therapeutic intervention for children with a myriad of exceptional problems, in order to minimize the potentially devastating psychosocial complications of exceptional problems.

chapter 9

A ONE-MONTH PEDIATRIC ROTATION IN DEVELOPMENTAL DISABILITIES

Mark L. Wolraich

Because of the many advances in pediatric technology, particularly in the area of neonatology, it is difficult to obtain the time to educate pediatric residents in the needs of exceptional children. Yet federal and state legislation for the handicapped has been enacted to guarantee the right of handicapped children to be educated and to reside in their home communities. As a consequence, pediatricians will be caring for an increasing number of exceptional children. All of us who are involved in pediatric training and who have an interest in exceptional children must utilize, to the utmost advantage, whatever time we are allotted in order to educate pediatricians in the needs of these children.

ELEMENTS OF THE ONE-MONTH ROTATION

A one-month mandatory rotation with time allotted in the second year of pediatric training provides a basis for implementing a curriculum for exceptional children. Using the 1-month rotation at the University of Iowa as an example, it is possible to demonstrate positive results from such a program. In designing our program, we were aware that past experience with similar rotations had suggested that there were several factors that made such rotations unpopular with the pediatric house staff. These rotations provided residents with too much observation but too little responsibility, too slow a pace to see change during the rotation, and too few activities that directly related to pediatric training. While popularity is not essential, the time pressures of pediatric residency will work to eliminate the program if the house staff does not perceive the rotation as worthwhile. Consequently, the pediatric 1-month rotation at the University of Iowa was designed to enhance the acceptability of such a rotation. Factors incorporated in the rotation format included: 1) maximizing resident responsibility and participation, 2) varying scheduling to compensate, to some degree, for the slow pace, 3) minimizing large group activities such as staffings, 4) maximizing one-to-one interactions between residents and staff, and 5) allowing one pediatric staff member the time to organize and teach the program.

Competency Based Objectives

Our rotation uses competency-based objectives to provide the basis for the pediatric training program content and evaluation. The American Board of Pediatrics has recently approached pediatric training utilizing competency-based objectives (*Foundations for Evaluating the Competency of Pediatricians,* 1974). Accordingly, the organization of the training curriculum has been divided into the five general areas of ability defined by the Board: 1) attitudes, 2) factual knowledge, 3) interpersonal skills, 4) technical skills, and 5) clinical judgment. Although the definition and evaluation of clinical judgment is still too subjective at this time, the four other general ability areas lend themselves well to adaptation for the development of a developmental disabilities curriculum. Each of these areas can be broken down into objectives, a plan of instruction, and can be evaluated. An outline of the actual curriculum developed at the University of Iowa is presented in the Appendix to this chapter.

An example of a competency-based objective designed to improve attitudes is objective "a" under "Attitudes" (see Appendix): "Improve the resident's ability to interact with developmentally disabled children in a comfortable and positive manner." Specifically, our aim was to have the residents comfortably communicate and play with developmentally disabled children, in medical and nonmedical settings, and thus develop a more positive attitude toward the children. An attempt was also made to help the resident have a realistic idea of what the potentials of developmentally disabled children are and what programs are important for their development.

To attain this objective, the rotation specifically attempted to maximize the residents' exposure to developmentally disabled children, particularly on a one-to-one basis. For example, the residents were made responsible for the day-to-day medical care of residential children within the hospital school facility. The residents also spent a period of time functioning as aides in a preschool classroom. Another project attempted to create an advocacy program with the adolescent population, but, due to administrative difficulties, that part of the plan has not been completed. Specific factual information relating to the legal rights and the sex education of the developmentally disabled was also provided.

Evaluating the Attitude Objective   The evaluation of the attitude objective consisted of three aspects. The first was a questionnaire called the Attitudes Towards Disabled Persons (ATDP) scale, which was developed by the Human Resources Center of Albertson, New York (Yuker, 1970). This questionnaire presents a series of 20 statements, such as, "Most disabled people worry a great deal." The respondent must react on a scale of 1 to 6 as to degree of agreement or disagreement. Low scores were an indication that the respondent perceived disabled persons as more different than the general population; high scores were an indication that the respondent perceived disabled persons as less different. The developers of the ATDP scale have interpreted perception of difference as an indication of negative attitudes toward disabled persons. However, the validity of this interpretation has not yet been demonstrated as it pertains to health professionals.

One weakness in the ATDP scale is that the word "disabled" is not defined. In a separate questionnaire, the residents were asked to choose the areas that they would include in the definition of "disabled." The residents selected from the physical, medical, emotional, social, and cultural areas. While virtually all of the residents included physical, medical, mental, and emotional in their responses, it is suspected that, particularly on the posttraining examination, they were thinking predominantly about the physically and mentally handicapped children with whom they dealt during their rotation in the Division of Developmental Disabilities.

The second aspect of evaluation related to the allocation of funds for developmental disabilities. The residents were asked what percentage of total funds they would allocate to institutions for the handicapped, to preschool developmental disabilities programs, to special schools for the developmentally disabled, and to preventive programs, if they were responsible for allocating funds on a state level.

A third aspect on which the residents were tested questioned whether or not they would put any qualifications for cardiac surgery for a ventricular septal defect on a child with Down's syndrome. We also plan a fourth area of evaluation, coding resident-child interactions with handicapped children by the use of a behavioral observation system.

The results of the ATDP are indicated in Table 1. The subjects were divided in half; the upper half was comprised of those residents who had the highest scores on their initial ATDP examination, or, according to the developers, perceived disabled people as least different. The lower half consisted of those residents with the lowest scores, or those who perceived disabled persons as most different. The mean score used for dividing the

Table 1. Attitudinal results — Attitudes Towards Disabled Persons Scale scores

Subjects	Mean[a]		Change	Sign test
	Pretest	Posttest		
Upper half on initial ATDP scores (N = 8)	84.4	73.1	−11.3	$p < 0.02$
Lower half on initial ATDP scores (N = 8)	76.4	71.3	− 5.1	NS

[a]Exam mean for nondisabled persons is 74.1.

group was derived by the developers through testing nonmedical personnel. Although change was not significant for residents in the low-scoring group, those in the high-scoring group did show a significant negative change when analyzed by the Wilcoxen Sign Test, i.e., they viewed disabled persons as more different.

If we use the test developers' interpretation of the results, it would appear that we had a negative attitudinal effect on the residents, i.e., the group that initially perceived disabled persons as less different perceived them as more different after the rotation. A second possible interpretation of the test scores is that the residents' perceptions of disabled persons had become more reality based at the end of the rotation. The residents whose scores were lower may have been thinking of the specific type of children they had been dealing with at the hospital school.

Despite the lack of change on the ATDP examination for the low-scoring group, there are other results that suggest we had some impact on the residents' attitudes toward the developmentally disabled. Table 2 presents the results of the responses to the question on allocation of monies for training programs in developmental disabilities. The group that perceived disabled persons as more different initially wanted to allocate more money for institutions than did the group that perceived disabled persons as less different. After their experiences on the rotation, however, both groups of residents decreased their interest in institutions. The lower-scoring group became more interested in developmental disability programs for preschool children by the end of the rotation.

Less ambiguous results were yielded by responses to the question relating to Down's syndrome. On the multiple choice question, seven of the eight residents in the group with the higher ATDP scores would have treated a ventricular septal defect without any qualifications, whereas only four out of eight of the lower-scoring residents would have done so. Two of these four residents changed their minds by the end of the rotation.

Table 2.   Allocation of monies for developmental disabilities programs[a]

Subjects	Institutions		Preschool programs		Special schools programs		Preventive programs	
	Pretest	Posttest	Pretest	Posttest	Pretest	Posttest	Pretest	Posttest
Upper half on initial ATDP scores (N=6)	25.8	23.3	29.2	27.5	17.5	22.5	29.2	26.7
Lower half on initial ATDP scores (N=6)	30.8	23.3	25.8	35.8	18.3	20.8	26.7	25.0

[a]The data represent percentages of total allocations.

111

Table 3.   Multiple choice exam results (N = 12)[a]

Section	Pretest	Posttest	Change	t test
Total	61.3	74.1	+ 12.8	$p < 0.001$
Developmental landmarks	69.1	74.5	+ 5.4	NS
Legal-ethical issues	68.0	70.7	+ 2.7	NS
Counseling	68.1	91.7	+ 23.6	$p < 0.01$
Cerebral palsy	31.7	66.7	+ 35.0	$p < 0.001$
Mental retardation	69.2	79.4	+ 10.2	$p < 0.01$
Spina bifida	58.3	76.9	+ 18.6	$p < 0.02$
School problems	46.1	60.8	+ 14.7	$p < 0.01$
Developmental assessment	56.7	66.7	+ 10.0	NS

[a]The results are the percentage of correct answers in each area.

Finally, the relationship between attitudes and the acquisition of information produced some interesting results. Scores on a multiple choice examination (see next section for details on this exam) for the high and low ATDP score groups revealed that the low group started out with slightly higher scores in terms of how much knowledge they had about developmentally disabled children. However, and most significant, they showed a much greater increase in their scores over the month than did the group with the higher scores on the ATDP. The difference in the change of scores between the high- and low-scoring groups was statistically significant.

Our results on attitude measures are certainly very preliminary and may change when the sample size is increased. Measuring attitudes is very complex, but is, nevertheless, necessary when considering training programs in developmental disabilities.

Improving Factual Knowledge

A second objective of the rotation program was to provide the residents with specific factual knowledge about developmentally disabled children. Didactic presentations, readings and discussion, and clinical experiences were the three modes of instruction. The readings consisted of articles in a bound notebook provided to the residents at the beginning of the month, which they were able to keep for the month's rotation. Designated books were easily accessible within the facility. The materials were divided into essential readings and readings for pursuing the subject in greater detail.

A 50-question multiple choice examination was given before and after the rotation. The examination was divided into the sections indicated in Table 3. Overall, significant improvement was noted in all areas except developmental landmarks, developmental assessment, and legal-ethical issues. Although it is clear that further improvement in instruction in developmental assessment is needed, the lack of effect on legal-ethical questions probably reflects the residents' prior ethical decisions, which are not easily changed. In addition, no attempt was made to teach the traditional developmental landmarks during the months' rotation, and the scores on the examination suggest that the residents already knew those landmarks fairly well before participating in the program. Although these results are preliminary due to the small number of residents and the fact that the pretest/posttest has certain limitations (see Chapter 11, this volume), they do suggest that the residents as a whole did read and retain most of the material provided. A strong attempt was made to ensure that the quantity of reading was not excessive and that the articles were pertinent to the residents' needs.

Improving Interpersonal Skills

A third important objective of the training program was to improve interpersonal skills. An emphasis was placed on counseling skills. Our use of the term *counseling* does not denote in-depth therapy as it usually does in the psychiatric or psychological literature. As it relates to pediatric residents, counseling means the ability to convey important information to parents and the ability to inform parents of catastrophic news. In a survey of the pediatric house staff at the University of Iowa, it was found that, while fairly specific training in pediatric interviewing is provided, training is not nearly as systematic as it relates to counseling skills. Since pediatric counseling situations are unpredictable, and invasion with observations and videotaping would be offensive, the pediatric rotation program staff developed the use of a simulated program with a parent counseling instructor. The opportunity was also provided for the residents to deal with actual families and to observe the approaches of clinicians within the facility. The parent counseling instructor had experience in interviewing skills and could simulate the role of a parent.

Three simulated situations were chosen: 1) a parent of a physically handicapped child of toddler age is seeking to establish medical supervision upon moving into a new area, 2) a parent of a newborn is to be told that the child has Down's syndrome, and 3) a parent is counseled who is resentful toward the physician's suggestion that the child is delayed and may need further evaluation. All the interviews were videotaped, and sessions were held after each taping to replay the tape with the parent counseling instructor and an experienced clinician present. Comments were made identifying the resident's strong points, and suggestions were made to improve techniques or to utilize alternative approaches.

In the program both pre- and post-counseling sessions are videotaped, and a behavior coding scale is currently being developed to evaluate the effects of the simulation. However, the reaction of the house staff has been very positive despite initial apprehensions of how well second year pediatric residents would respond to the simulated sessions. Subjectively, it should be noted that there seemed to be improvement in the majority of the residents between the pre- and post-taping.

SUMMARY

In summary, we feel that it is important to carefully utilize the training time available in pediatric residency programs and that this is best done by building from a groundwork of competency-based objectives. The material presented in this chapter provides preliminary results of such an undertaking. In taking the time and effort required for such programs, there is the added benefit of demonstrating a potentially effective training approach to other areas of pediatric training.

REFERENCES

American Board of Pediatrics, Inc. 1974. Foundations for Evaluating the Competency of Pediatricians. Chicago: American Board of Pediatrics, Inc.

Yuker, H. E. 1970. The Measurement of Attitudes Towards Disabled Persons. Albertson, N.Y.: Human Resource Center.

APPENDIX

Currriculum Outline for Developmental Disabilities Rotation for Pediatric Residents

A. ATTITUDES

　I. *Attitudes Towards Developmentally Disabled Children*

　　a. *Objective: Improve the resident's ability to interact with* developmentally disabled children in a comfortable and positive manner.

　　Specifically:

　　1. The resident should be able to talk and play with the children without being uncomfortable. His/her conversation should be appropriate for the particular child.

　　2. The resident should have a realistic idea of what presently can be done for these children and why the programs are important.

　　3. The resident should have a positive attitude towards developmentally disabled children.

　　b. *Plan of instruction:*

　　1. Maximum exposure clinically to developmentally disabled children, particularly on a one-to-one basis.

　　(a) Have the resident participate in the preschool class setting for one hour.

(b)   Make morning rounds of the residential hospital school children.
2. Factual (presented by reading and discussion).
   (a)   Legal rights of the developmentally disabled.
   (b)   Sex education of the developmentally disabled.
c. *Evaluation:*
   1. Written questions.
      (a)   ATDP exam.
      (b)   Question on the allocation of funds for developmental disabilities.
      (c)   Videotaped resident-child interaction coded by behavioral criteria.
   2. Subjective evaluation by staff members.

II. *Attitudes Towards and Use of Allied Health Professionals*
   a. *Objectives:*   The resident should have an understanding of the functioning of Allied Health Professionals so that he/she is able to make appropriate referrals in order to provide optimal care for patients.
      1. He/she should be able to describe what Allied Health Professionals do. The Allied Health Professionals included in our program will be:
         (a)   Psychologist.
         (b)   Speech Pathologist.
         (c)   Dentist.
         (d)   Social Worker.
         (e)   Occupational Therapist.
         (f)   Physical Therapist.
         (g)   Pediatric Nurse Practitioner.
         (h)   Public Health Nurse.
      2. He/she should be able to describe what types of problems should be referred to the Allied Health Professionals named above.
      3. He/she should be able to know what information would be helpful to those Allied Health Professionals named above.
      4. He/she should know what information the Allied Health Professionals named above can provide.
      5. He/she should be able to determine the competency of the Allied Health Professionals named above based on qualifications of training.
      6. He/she should be able to communicate freely with the Allied Health Professionals.
      7. He/she should be receptive to suggestions the Allied

Health Professionals can make towards the resident's evaluation and management of developmentally disabled children.

b. *Plan of instruction:*
1. Factual information — The resident will be provided with a booklet of information about the Allied Health Professionals named above which addresses itself to the information stated in the Educational Objectives.
2. Clinical exposure.
   (a) The resident will see various Allied Health Professionals in their diagnostic roles as part of participation in the clinics, both in Hospital School and Child Development Clinic, as well as other parts of his/her program.
   (b) The resident will spend at least one therapy session with an Occupational Therapist, Physical Therapist, and Speech Pathologist. During these sessions he/she will have the opportunity to both observe and help out with the particular therapy with which that professional is engaged.

c. *Evaluation:*
1. Written exam with questions that address the factual information that is provided.
2. Subjective evaluations by those Allied Health Professionals who deal with the resident. They will be asked to judge ability to communicate with them.

B. FACTUAL KNOWLEDGE
  I. *Developmental Assessment*
    a. *Objectives:*
1. To be able to state with 80% accuracy a basic list of developmental landmarks useful in following normal children.
2. Be able to describe the different developmental exams stating their:
   (a) Use.
   (b) Format.
   (c) How standardized.
   (d) Limitations.
   (e) Reliability.
   (Exams will include Gesell, Bayley, Cattell, Denver, Stanford-Binet, and Wechsler.)
3. Be able to list causes of developmental delay.*

*See IV b and c for plan of instruction and evaluation.

II. *Physically Handicapping Conditions*
  a. *Objectives:*
    1. Should be able to state with regard to cerebral palsy:
      (a) Cause and pathophysiology.
      (b) Types.
      (c) Prognoses.
      (d) Types of therapy available.
    2. Should be able to state with regard to meningomyelocele:
      (a) Effects of the defects.
      (b) Causes and risk to parents.
      (c) Prognosis and treatments available.*
III. *Mental Retardation*
  a. *Objectives:*
    1. Should be able to state classifications.
    2. Should be able to state major causes and prognosis for each entity.
    3. Should be able to state types of community programs available and current trends.*
IV. *School Problems*
  a. *Objectives:*
    1. Should be able to state definition of minimal brain dysfunction and state difficulties with its definition.
    2. Should be able to state differing viewpoints of diagnosis and treatment of hyperactivity.
    3. Should be able to state definition of learning disabilities.
    4. Should be able to state controversial forms of therapy available for hyperactivity and explain basis of controversies for each form of therapy.
  b. *Plan of instruction for all above-stated factual areas:*
    1. Didactic presentations.
    2. Readings and discussions.
    3. Informally as part of clinical experience.
  c. *Evaluation:* Written exam.

C. INTERPERSONAL SKILLS
  I. *Counseling of Families*
    a. *Objective:* The resident should be able to counsel parents of handicapped children.
      1. He/she should have several counseling techniques at their disposal such as use of empathy.
      2. He/she should have an understanding of most common handicapping conditions as to effect on family,

prognosis, and therapeutic resources that are available.

   3. He/she should know the usual reaction of parents to having a child with significant mental or physical deficits.

  b. *Plan of instruction:*

    1. Simulated situation to be videotaped with feedback.

    2. Observations of the approaches of the various pediatric staff here.

    3. Opportunity to counsel families with feedback if possible.

  c. *Evaluation (Pre-Post):*

    1. Simulated parent conference videotaped with analysis of:

      (a) Empathetic statements made.

      (b) Extent of determining both medical and psychosocial concerns.

      (c) Ability to educate parents to the disability, prognosis, and treatment.

    2. Written exam.

D. TECHNICAL SKILLS

  I. *Developmental Assessment*

    a. *Objective:* The resident should be able, using printed information, to evaluate the developmental status of a child five years or under to a degree sufficient for screening purposes. He/she should know techniques to help the child cooperate and he/she should demonstrate the ability to present the tasks in a consistent acceptable way.

    b. *Plans of instruction:*

      1. Didactic presentation of history, content, and methods of developmental assessment.

      2. Presentation of skills needed to properly administer assessment scale.

      3. Videotaping of residents carrying out assessments with feedback.

    c. *Evaluation:*

      1. Videotaping of assessment on a child.

      2. Written exam.

  II. *Assessment of Motorically Handicapped Children*

    a. *Objective:* The resident should be able to determine the motoric abilities of handicapped children so that he/she can:

      1. Make appropriate referrals to other specialists or allied health professionals.
      2. Determine a categorical diagnosis if possible.
      3. Be able to get some idea of prognosis.
b. *Plan of instruction:*
      1. Didactic presentation.
      2. Direct patient contact in the diagnostic and therapeutic situation under supervision.
c. *Evaluation: Subjective evaluation of staff supervising the resident.*

chapter 10

A THREE-MONTH RESIDENCY CURRICULUM IN CHILD DEVELOPMENT AND HANDICAPPED CHILDREN

Forrest C. Bennett

Pediatric residents at the University of Washington in Seattle receive the majority of their training in child development and exceptional children at the Child Development and Mental Retardation Center, a large University Affiliated Facility within the Department of Pediatrics. Every 3 months, 3 PL-2 residents come to the Center, which accommodates a total of 12 residents each academic year. The University of Washington Pediatric Residency Program currently includes about 14 PL-2 house officers; thus, almost all residents in the program receive at least 3 months of concentrated training on the recognition and care of young exceptional children. While at the Center, their experience is guided primarily by a developmental pediatrician with subspecialty training in child development and handicapped children. They also closely interact with one or two developmental disability fellows who participate in the teaching program.

GOALS AND PROGRAM DESCRIPTION

There are three major goals for that segment of the pediatric house officers' education that are provided at the Child Development Center: 1) a firm foundation in normal child development, 2) a broad experience in the varieties of abnormal child development, and 3) an introduction to the interdisciplinary process. These three objectives are intimately intertwined in the residents' experiences and responsibilities at the Center. The skills of identifying and assessing atypical development arise from an adequate appreciation and understanding of the wide variations of normal development. And, perhaps of greatest importance for future pediatricians, these abilities and sensitivities are learned within a framework necessitating close interaction with the full range of child development specialists and fostering interdisciplinary communication and decision-making.

The pediatric resident spends 2 days each week in our Well Child Clinic (see Table 1). This clinic is the cornerstone for appreciating the dynamic aspects of normal child development. Children are seen at frequent intervals from birth through adolescence under the guidance of a developmental pediatrician and with the close consulting support of a variety of specialists in related disciplines, particularly social work and nutrition. The pediatric resident, as in no other ambulatory setting in his/her overall program, is both allowed and encouraged to spend extra time (45–60 minutes) with families at these visits. Interviewing skills are evaluated (with the availability of videotape critique), anticipatory counseling is encouraged, and the concept and methods of periodic developmental assessments are presented. Residents become familiar with the appropriate use of widely accepted developmental screening tools, including a parent questionnaire, the Alpern-Boll Developmental Profile, and the Denver Developmental Screening Test.

A Developmental Perspective

A philosophy of so-called "routine" well child care is put forth that makes the detection of potential growth, developmental, and behavioral aberrations at least as important as the detection of unrecognized, asymptomatic physical disease. Accordingly, a lecture series on related developmental topics (e.g., infant bonding and attachment, infant crying, separation anxiety, sleep disturbances, stages of equilibrium and disequilibrium, language development and speech dysfluency, and school readiness) plus introductory readings in developmental theory (Piaget, Erikson, Skinner, Gesell) complement the clinical experience. Observations of children in groups are encouraged, and a wide range of community preschool (Head Start, Montessori, Bank Street Model) and school-age (self-contained, open concept, accelerated) programs are available. The Well Child Clinic exists at our Center because of our strong conviction that residents must compare and contrast normal and abnormal child development together, on both a theoretical and practical level, for both types of development to be adequately learned.

Table 1.   Pediatric residents' basic program at the Child Development and Mental Retardation Center

Time of day	Day of week				
	Monday	Tuesday	Wednesday	Thursday	Friday
Morning	Child Study Clinic	Child Study Clinic	NICU Follow-up Clinic	Grand Rounds/ Well Child Clinic	Well Child Clinic
Afternoon	Child Study Clinic	Behavioral Disorders Clinic/Neurology	NICU Follow-up Clinic	Well Child Clinic	Well Child Clinic

Neonatal Intensive Care and Follow-up

The pediatric resident spends 1 day each week in our Neonatal Intensive Care Unit (NICU) Follow-up Clinic. This clinic bridges the gap between normal and abnormal development in a select, high risk population. The development of the smallest and sickest survivors of the University Hospital Neonatal Intensive Care Unit (including all infants with hyaline membrane disease, all with a birth weight of 1500 grams or less, all with neonatal central nervous system infection, and most with neonatal seizures or suspected intracranial hemorrhage) is followed closely by pediatricians, physical therapists, psychologists, and audiologists.

The resident functions in two alternating roles in this clinic. Some of the time the resident is the pediatrician for the child's annual review of past and present physical problems. At other times, the resident observes and participates in the physical therapy evaluation of motor development and becomes familiar with the philosophy and administration of current psychological tests as they apply to the cognitive, language, and social development of premature children. Particularly useful as adjuncts to traditional neurological procedures are the physical therapy techniques of early identification of motor disorders and the methods of teaching parents to handle infants with these disorders.

The resident often has the opportunity to follow-up infants and parents he/she cared for in the NICU. He/she learns to appreciate the frequently poor correlation between specific neonatal events and developmental outcome. Moreover, the resident is heartened by 1000 gram infants with numerous adverse neonatal complications who develop appropriately and is saddened and puzzled by infants with relatively benign neonatal courses who develop cerebral palsy. More than any other single developmental disorder, the resident experiences the dynamic, changing natural history and the wide variation in severity of this static encephalopathy as it is still frequently encountered in this clinic.

Child Study Clinic

The pediatric resident spends 1½ days of each week in our Child Study Clinic. This clinic provides exposure to children of all ages with the full spectrum of developmental disabilities. Typical problems handled by the resident include: mental deficiency of varying degrees of severity, questions of autism or "autistic" behaviors, cerebral palsy, recognized and unrecognized multiple malformation syndromes, specific language disability (developmental dysphasia) with near normal cognition, school learning disability, special sensory deficits (deaf and/or blind children), and environmental deprivation with abuse and neglect. The resident particularly must wrestle with the concepts of developmental delay and mental retardation with his/her families and must determine which is most appropriate in each individual case; thus balancing the creation of unrealistic expectations against the devastation of withdrawing all hope. The resident also experiences the personal and parental frustration of the many children whose mental deficiency remains unexplained (idiopathic) even after a thorough medical search.

Children seen in this clinic for diagnostic and developmental evaluation are referred from a variety of sources: parents, physicians, preschool and school teachers, therapists, and social agencies. The resident is responsible for their physical and developmental examination while working with members from other disciplines on a child development team. Questions pertaining to the etiology of a handicap must be explored, and thus the need for a thorough prenatal history, perinatal history, developmental history, and family history is emphasized. Residents are encouraged to follow a child through the entire evaluative process. In so doing, they become acquainted with the strengths and weaknesses of the commonly used psychological measures (including intelligence test controversies), they learn to separate language into its receptive and expressive components, and they determine appropriate referral criteria for speech therapy. They are also exposed to the theories and terminology of occupational therapy and are introduced to the different types of special education programs available in urban and rural school districts under the Education for All Handicapped Children Act, Public Law 94-142.

The resident is expected to be the case manager for a number of children. In this role, he/she learns to deal with the community resources that serve exceptional children, as well as their referral patterns. The resident is thrust into the usually new and uncomfortable position of directing the team conference that synthesizes the case. Here, separated from the customary medical support system, the resident is one of many child development professionals, and he/she must practice interdisciplinary communication. The resident has the responsibility for interpreting the complex and sensitive results of the evaluation for the parents, and he/she is guided in counseling techniques applicable to many chronic handicapping conditions. This informing process often includes genetic counseling as well.

Behavioral Disorders Clinic

The pediatric resident spends 1 half-day each week in our Behavioral Disorders Clinic. This clinic provides a unique opportunity to formulate behavioral intervention strategies, to utilize learning theory, and to teach parenting practices in difficult cases of disordered family functioning. It is directed by a pediatrician with a background in mental retardation who currently has a private practice devoted exclusively to behavioral and developmental pediatrics.

The clinic provides the resident with an alternative model to the single diagnostic evaluation by a large team. Here, the resident is presented young children with behavioral and, often, learning problems, and is primarily responsible, under the director's guidance, for assessing the difficulties, instituting a behavioral program if indicated, obtaining appropriate consultation (i.e., psychology, psychiatry, or speech pathology), and seeing the family in follow-up at frequent intervals. The purpose of this clinic is to teach the resident an approach to these common home and school problems that can be applied to a primary care setting. There is ample exposure to areas of current controversy, such as the concept of minimal brain dysfunction (MBD), the opportunity to weigh stimulant drug therapy against strictly behavioral techniques, and the chance to observe these children in the classroom to get a better understanding of the teacher's complaints.

Ancillary Opportunities and Specialty Clinics

In addition to the pediatric residents' basic program at the Center, there are numerous ancillary opportunities and specialty clinics available. The resident can spend some limited time in those of his/her choosing during the initial 3 months at the Center and then can return for intensive 1-month electives in individual clinics. A particularly unique opportunity is afforded by our Experimental Education Unit, housed within the Center. Here, the resident can observe, and occasionally participate in, model educational programs for handicapped children. These programs include a comprehensive birth-to-6 years learning program for Down's syndrome children, a communication disorders preschool for children with language disabilities, a preschool for children with severe behavior problems, an early elementary school program for learning disabled children, and a program for severely and profoundly retarded children, including children with diagnoses of autism. The resident may on occasion evaluate a child with a developmental disability in our Child Study Clinic, recommend this child for a program in the Experimental Education Unit, and then have opportunity to follow the child's progress in the classroom.

Specialty clinics are available at the Center in dysmorphology, biochemical disorders, phenylketonuria, and the Prader-Willi syndrome. A Pediatric Neurology Clinic meets 1 day per week, and all residents spend some time in this clinic with a neurologist who has an extensive background in mental retardation. Related clinics in birth defects, medical genetics, rehabilitation medicine, and child psychiatry for exceptional children are available at other locations in the Residency Program.

Table 2. Comparison of University of Washington program with other programs on the American Board of Pediatrics written examination, 1971-1975

Section of exam	Mean[a]		University of Washington rank
	University of Washington	All other programs	
Newborn	522	473	26.5
Metabolic disorders	523	472	27.5
Growth and development	542	443	7.0
Infectious disease	515	466	31.0
General	514	470	32.0
Total test	527	458	16.0

[a] n = 240

Evaluation

Residents are asked to critically evaluate all of their clinical experiences at the Center upon completion of the 3-month program. The three features most consistently given positive appraisal are the teaching of the nonmedical child development professionals (especially psychology, speech pathology, and physical therapy), the experience of high risk neonatal followup, and the availability of a developmental pediatrician with the time to help synthesize their many experiences. Negative aspects mentioned include insufficient teaching about exceptional children and their needs by program physicians, other disciplines overestimating their knowledge and sophistication in developmental areas, and the inefficiencies of team functioning. Thus, the residents are repeatedly saying that they have not had much experience with exceptional children and that they welcome all the teaching help they can get.

Residents are contacted by mail several years after completion of their training program and asked to evaluate their proficiency in dealing with exceptional children and the frequency with which they utilize such expertise in their practice. Over 85% of those pediatricians returning the questionnaire felt that: 1) the skills gained at the Center are very relevant to their current practice, 2) the interdisciplinary approach was helpful, and 3) their overall understanding of and empathy for handicapped children and adults was increased. In fact, developmental pediatrics is one of the more common fellowship choices of those University of Washington residents who pursue subspecialty training. For example, of the 14 pediatric residents who completed the training program in 1973 (myself included), 4 of us completed fellowship training in the area of child development and handicapped children.

Finally, University of Washington residents have had consistently high scores on the Growth and Development Section of the American Board of Pediatrics written examination when compared with national norms and have ranked near the top among pediatric programs for this Section (Table 2). We hope that these results may, in part, reflect the importance given to developmental pediatrics by our overall residency program and, more specifically, the training received at the Child Development Center.

chapter 11

AN EVALUATION STRATEGY FOR PEDIATRIC ROTATIONS ON THE NEEDS OF EXCEPTIONAL CHILDREN

H. Burtt Richardson, Jr., and Michael J. Guralnick

There is general agreement that experience with exceptional children and the professionals from various disciplines who serve their developmental needs is an important component in pediatric education. Of equal importance is the systematic evaluation of these experiences. In spite of this agreement, our search for curricula incorporating this experience, particularly those that have objectively evaluated results of such curriculum segments, has revealed only a few published examples (see Chapter 1, this volume). Given the importance of systematic evaluation in answering basic questions about any curriculum segment, (e.g., "Is it worth our time and effort?" and "How can we change it to make it more effective?"), we present in this chapter an application of certain fundamental concepts of evaluation to situations involving pediatric residency rotations.

DESCRIPTION OF THE CURRICULUM

Our efforts toward designing an evaluation strategy were carried out in the context of a program providing a short-term exposure of pediatric residents to exceptional children in a preschool setting (see Richardson and Guralnick, 1978; Richardson, Guralnick, and Tupper, 1978). The experience for the residents consisted of activities for 1 half-day per week for a

This work was supported in part by Grant OEG-GOO-77-00705 from the United States Office of Education, Bureau of Education for the Handicapped.

129

4-week period at the preschool. Second or third year residents were available each month from September through June (the months that the preschool operated) and the curriculum to be evaluated was based on that 12-hour experience.

The pediatric residents observed and interacted with handicapped children and their parents at a model demonstration preschool. Resident activities were carefully specified, organized in modular form, and related to a series of objectives, such as: "Gain sensitivity to and comfort with individual handicapped children," or "Gain knowledge of the terminology of special education." (See Richardson, Guralnick, and Tupper, 1978, for further details.) Active participation of the residents included working directly with selected handicapped children, as well as interviews and other interactions with the teachers, the speech therapist, the social worker, and related child development professionals. These activities were supplemented by providing a number of videotapes, slide tapes, selected readings, didactic presentations, and exemplary medical, psychological, educational, social work, and hearing and speech reports.

EVALUATION APPROACHES

From the field of evaluation we can extract two dimensions that are particularly relevant to our evaluation strategy. It is not that other concepts such as sampling and generalizability are not germane, but for purposes of this discussion only two dimensions are emphasized here. As illustrated in Figure 1, the first dimension of the evaluation strategy is that of the degree of objectivity of our data. In many instances we must rely on the subjective impressions of participants to assess our effectiveness even though the ability of individuals to observe and accurately report their impressions is always of concern. Nevertheless, data in this form often provide essential information, especially at early stages of an investigation. Of course, achieving a highly reliable objective evaluation is generally more desirable, but even highly objective data are subject to criticism, such as that regarding the validity of the constructs to which the observations are related (see Johnson and Bolstad, 1973).

The first question we needed to answer in our program was: "Do the residents say the experience is valuable?" This, of course, would yield subjective results, but it is in fact an important issue for the training program director. Accordingly, during the program's first year, at the end of each rotation we listed each objective and asked the residents to use a 9-point scale to assess whether each objective was important, whether the program was effective in carrying out the objectives, and whether the resident had gained competence and confidence in the area of each objective over the course of the 4-week period. In general, the results indicated that the various objectives were seen as important, the program was moder-

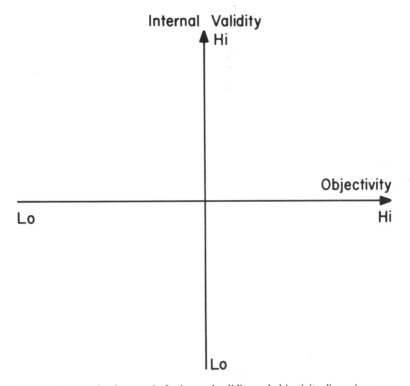

Figure 1.   An evaluation matrix for internal validity and objectivity dimensions.

ately effective in carrying out the objectives, and the residents perceived a gain in their competence and confidence in each area over the course of the training period.

Such an evaluation of the program, although important, certainly lacks objectivity, but it further lacks internal validity — our second dimension (Figure 1). Internal validity, in this instance, refers to the degree to which we can be assured that the results are attributable to the impact of the program or the curriculum rather than to other factors. That is, the residents might have provided their positive impressions for a host of reasons other than those related to the true effectiveness of the program in bringing about the desired changes. Unfortunately, the designs used most frequently in the evaluation of educational programs are case studies (posttest only without a control group) and pretest/posttest comparisons. In the case study approach, there is, of course, no assurance that the curriculum accounts for the results obtained in the posttest. It is less frequently recognized, however, that pretest/posttest comparisons, even with a control group, are often weak in internal validity because the pretest can strongly influence the results of the posttest.

Design for Evaluation

Accordingly, during the second year of our program, we not only introduced a more objective measure of change (a posttest), but we also sought
to utilize an experimental design that permitted us to be more confident
that any changes we obtained were attributable directly to the curriculum
(Richardson and Guralnick, 1978). Our efforts were complicated by the
fact that we were faced with the situation of having 18 second and third
year residents scheduled for 1- or 2-month elective periods evenly
throughout the school year, all of whom expected and indeed, from our
point of view, needed an exposure to handicapped children in a preschool
setting. Selecting experimental and control groups in this situation was a
challenge, but we ultimately chose a modification of the posttest only with
control group design (see Campbell and Stanley, 1962).

Our method was to divide the 10-month period from September
through June into five sequential experimental periods. As indicated in
Figure 2, members of the experimental group were scheduled to participate in the program during the months of September, November, Janu-
ary, March, and May, whereas control group members were scheduled
during October, December, February, April, and June. The majority of
the 18 residents were assigned to psychiatry for 2-month blocks integrated
with an outpatient experience during the five time periods. The remainder
were assigned to physical medicine and rehabilitation. Whether a resident
spent the 4 half-days at the demonstration preschool program during the
first month (that is, was a member of the experimental group) or the second month (control group member) was determined randomly.

In this manner, for example, two residents would have just completed the program (experimental group) and would receive a posttest. At
the same time, or the following week, the next group of two residents
(control group) who were about to participate in the program would receive the same test. By repeating this sequence every 2 months, additional
members were added to each group, thereby generating an adequate subject population to serve as a basis for assessing the impact of the program.

Of course, with the exception of the authors, no one else was aware
of the experimental design. To the control group, the evaluation appeared
to be a traditional pretest/posttest comparison measuring their own
change over the course of the month. Although we were thereby permitted
a pretest/posttest comparison as well, the critical comparison was between the control group and the experimental group.

Assessment Instruments: Objectivity

We attempted to obtain data that had a high degree of objectivity. Accordingly, instead of relying on subjective impressions of change exclusively, we designed a variety of instruments to measure the acquisition of:

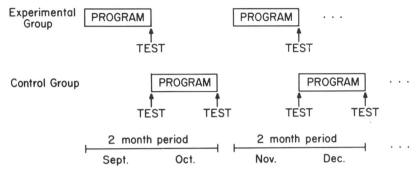

Figure 2.   Two 2-month block periods of the experimental design to improve internal validity compatible with pediatric rotation schedules.

1) knowledge about handicapping conditions and their management, 2) skills in describing the specific behaviors of handicapped children in the context of environmental contingencies, 3) attitudes toward handicapped children as judged by the positivity of behavioral descriptions, and 4) clinical judgment in counseling parents and selecting further studies.

The knowledge component consisted of a series of multiple choice questions relating to readings and didactic sessions. The remaining components (skill, attitude, and clinical judgment) were all derived from a series of open-ended questions based on a videotape of a handicapped child. The following situation was presented (see Richardson and Guralnick, 1978):

> You are the pediatrician of a preschool child who has learning handicaps. You have an opportunity to visit the child's preschool and observe her behavior briefly in both the classroom and in a free-play setting (to be observed on videotape).

A brief videotape of the handicapped child interacting in these two situations was then shown. Immediately after the viewing of the videotape, the resident was asked to answer the following questions: (a) "Please write below the brief entry you would make in your records about your observations," (b) "Please write below what you would tell your patient's parents about what you observed in her school," and (c) "Please list the studies, consultations, and/or reports you would obtain (or would have obtained) in your evaluation of your patient."

The skill of residents in making specific behavioral observations was assessed by a content analysis of each phrase, clause, or sentence in questions (a) and (b). The use of statements containing labels, such as retarded, aphasic, or autistic, anchored one end of the scale, whereas specific statements of behavior, particularly those involving environmental events and relationships, anchored the other end.

Table 1. Comparisons between experimental and control group scores for three major dimensions derived from test to evaluate pediatric training program

Dimensions	Experimental group	Control group
Knowledge		
I	4.44^a	3.00
II^b	67.00^a	0.00
Skills-Specificity	6.78	6.11
Attitude-Positivity		
Question (a)	6.44^a	3.56
Question (b)	6.11	3.55

Richardson, H. B., and Guralnick, M. J. 1978. Pediatric residents and young handicapped children: The systematic evaluation of a curriculum. *Journal of Medical Education,* 53. Reprinted by permission.

$^a p < 0.05.$

^{b}Analysis is based on the Fisher Exact Probability Test; data consist of percentage correct for total group.

The residents' attitudes toward handicapped children was measured along a positivity-negativity dimension also obtained from a content analysis of questions (a) and (b). Clinical judgment was assessed by analyzing and categorizing the nature of advice, consultation, and reports requested.

By utilizing assessment instruments in this form, we were able to obtain reliability estimates for each measure. For example, reliability of the content analysis for specificity and positivity of the statements ranged from 80%-90%, as judged by independent raters.

The Program's Impact

Results of the comparison between the nine residents in the experimental group and the nine residents in the control group are presented in Table 1. As indicated, the knowledge dimension was divided into two components, both of which showed a significant superiority in favor of the experimental group. However, there were no significant differences between the two groups in terms of skills in specifying the handicapped child's behavior or in the clinical judgment in the selection of further clinical studies. Closer inspection of the data suggested that the failure to obtain differences in clinical judgment may well have been due to the insensitivity of the measure, probably reflecting a ceiling effect. For the specificity measure, the curriculum did not appear to transmit the necessary skills despite the fact that the teaching staff described the youngsters' behavior in this way.

The most interesting finding of the study was a significant difference in attitude as reflected by the positivity of residents in describing the handicapped child's behavior. On question (a) there was a clearly significant difference in the residents' description of the child's behavior on the videotape, and a similar analysis of question (b) fell just short of the required level of significance.

CONCLUSIONS

Gratifying as these limited significant differences between the experimental and control groups were, it was the design of the study and its ability to enhance the degree of objectivity and internal validity of our evaluation, even within the time and scheduling constraints posed by a busy pediatric residency, that we feel were of greater importance. Certainly, the major advantage of this type of design is that members of the control group are not deprived of participation in the curriculum but have to wait only a brief period of time prior to their involvement. A major limitation imposed by the method is that only short-term effects of the curriculum can be measured. The control group is exposed to the curriculum prior to an opportunity for any longer term follow-up. However, the merits of the technique, in particular the increase in the internal validity of experimental comparisons that can be achieved, are notable. Furthermore, this design is especially useful for assessing the effects of new components of a specific curriculum or for determining the effective ingredients of a multicomponent program.

The final test of a program's effectiveness, of course, is the long-term impact of the curriculum and, specifically, its generalizability to pediatrician behavior outside of the experimental setting. Such tests of external validity are beyond the scope and budgets of many pediatric training programs, but such limitations should not discourage training program directors and others responsible for specific components of the residents' curriculum from carrying on evaluation with as high a degree of objectivity and internal validity as the particular situation will allow.

REFERENCES

Campbell, D. T., and Stanley, J. C. 1962. Experimental and Quasiexperimental Designs for Research. Chicago: Rand McNally and Co.

Johnson, S. M., and Bolstad, O. D. 1973. Methodological issues in naturalistic observation: Some problems and solutions for field research. In L. A. Hamerlynck, L. D. Handy and E. J. Mash (Eds.), Critical Issues in Research and Practice: Proceedings of the Fourth Banff International Conference in Behavior Modification. Champaign, Ill.: Research Press.

Richardson, H. B., and Guralnick, M. J. 1978. Pediatric residents and young handicapped children: The systematic evaluation of a curriculum. Journal of Medical Education, 53, 487–492.

Richardson, H. B., Guralnick, M. J., and Tupper, D. B. 1978. Training pediatricians for effective involvement with handicapped preschool children and their families. Mental Retardation, 16, 3–7.

chapter 12

A FELLOWSHIP PROGRAM ON THE NEEDS OF EXCEPTIONAL CHILDREN

Arnold J. Capute and Pasquale J. Accardo

The current generation of physician leaders in the field of developmental disabilities is mostly self-taught. The next generation of developmentalists will benefit greatly from exposure to formal developmental training as it is now being organized in University Affiliated Facilities and other post-doctoral level pediatric fellowship training programs. Indeed, with the exponential increase of disability related information in medical and paramedical areas, it is doubtful whether physicians can attain sufficient competence to function as leaders, teachers, and advocates in the field of chronic handicapping conditions without such specialty training.

The training program in Developmental Pediatrics at the John F. Kennedy Institute of the Johns Hopkins University School of Medicine has as its goal the training of Board eligible or certified pediatricians in the area of developmental disabilities (mental retardation, cerebral palsy, learning disabilities, autism, hearing and visual impairments, and convulsive disorders when associated with the above). The trainees become expert in the transdisciplinary[1] approach to the evaluation and management

---

The preparation of this chapter was supported in part through Project 917, Maternal and Child Health Service, United States Department of Health, Education and Welfare. The manuscript was typed by Linda Chandlee, Craig Daley, and Karen Torbit.

[1]Since the terms are often loosely interchanged, a brief note of clarification appears to be in order. *Multidisciplinary* implies that a child has been evaluated by several specialists with differing training backgrounds and frequently conflicting theoretical models to interpret the same developmental phenomena. Their intercommunication may be restricted to an exchange of written reports and may be hampered by a high degree of professional jargon; when they do meet in committee, their common goal of helping the child contributes to keeping the confusion and bloodshed to a minimum. *Interdisciplinary* suggests that the different

of handicapped children by learning to use the tools, the techniques, and the methodologies employed by the various medical and nonmedical disciplines in patient management. The medical specialties of pediatrics, pediatric neurology, neurophysiology, electroencephalography, child psychiatry, genetics, pediatric surgery, neurosurgery, neonatology, ophthalmology, otolaryngology, dermatology, orthopedic surgery, and physiatry (rehabilitation medicine) are included in the program as well as nonmedical disciplines such as child psychology, special education, audiology, speech pathology, physical therapy, occupational therapy, biochemistry, social services, nursing, ethology, anthropology, psycholinguistics, history of childhood, and medical ethics.

The training program requires 2 to 3 years following completion of a 3-year approved residency in pediatrics. In broadest outline, the program includes: 1) 6 months of inpatient service, 2) 6 months of outpatient service, 3) 4 months of pediatric neurology, and 4) 4-month rotations on two of the following: child psychiatry, perinatology, EEG laboratory, a genetics and biochemical elective, and other appropriate experiences that will enhance the trainee's evaluative and management skills. (The optional third year may be used to obtain an M.P.H. degree or pursue specialized research interests.) A brief description of the purpose of each of these rotations follows.

THE PROGRAM

Inpatient Rotation

The John F. Kennedy Institute maintains an inpatient teaching unit of forty beds. An admissions committee composed of representatives from each of the core disciplines selects patients to serve as model cases for both medical and nonmedical trainees. The patient is initially evaluated through a neurodevelopmental history and examination performed by the pediatric fellow. The fellow then follows the patient through the remainder of the evaluation and observes the management process so that he/she learns to supervise and coordinate not only the evaluation, but the

---

professionals actually succeed in communicating to the other professionals on the team the relevance of their varying perspectives to the understanding of the whole child; contrary to general opinion, the success of this communication is not due to good will, personality traits and temperament, or the use of paucisyllabic English, but is the result of a prolonged (i.e., measured in years rather than months) training experience in an interdisciplinary setting. *Transdisciplinary* describes the ability of professionals to cross over and function effectively in areas outside their primary specialization. In general, multidisciplinary teams are common, well-functioning interdisciplinary teams are much less common, and true transdisciplinary functioning is exceedingly rare. The handicapped child for his/her part needs the services of multiple specialists; the specialists, on their part, do not always succeed in ironing out their interprofessional rivalries in getting their act together.

therapy program as well. It is essential that the pediatric trainee observe nonmedical professionals as they evaluate the child and the family in order to become familiar with their techniques for assessment and their use in the design of an habilitation program. As soon as the evaluation process is completed, there is a steering conference (the afternoon of the second hospital day) in which all of the disciplines discuss their findings and recommendations. Projected therapeutic goals are clearly defined and outlined so that each of the involved disciplines has a clear picture of the child's prognosis. After the steering conference, the parents are counseled with regard to the results of the evaluation, and the management program is thoroughly discussed so that the parents can assume an active role. Periodic follow-up conferences are planned in which the participating disciplines discuss the progress of the therapy program. Necessary alterations of the habilitation program are implemented so as to maximize the child's functioning. The inpatient service contributes significantly to the overall training program since it gives the trainee an opportunity to work very closely with other disciplines for long periods of time in the follow-up of children who are in medium- to long-term therapy programs. (See Figure 1 for the sequence of events for this process.)

On the inpatient service, the pediatric fellow admits approximately 3 new patients a week and carries an average caseload of 10 patients through the multidisciplinary management phase. Daily 8 a.m. rounds are held at which a single case is reviewed in depth from a developmental pediatric perspective; physical and neurodevelopmental findings are demonstrated by the attending physician in charge. Since this usually occurs prior to the steering conference, the sensitivity of this evaluation can be measured against the more detailed multidisciplinary assessment. Weekly X-ray rounds utilize the films on the inpatients for a teaching conference in the Department of Pediatric Radiology and all inpatients receive a detailed ophthalmologic examination at weekly eye rounds.

A series of 5 p.m. lectures is repeated every 3 weeks (to match the rotation of the medical students and residents). The first 2 weeks cover the core curriculum (see Accardo and Capute, 1979) of mental retardation, cerebral palsy, learning disabilities, and related psychological, neurological, and biochemical subjects. The topics for the last week will vary during the year to reflect the special clinical or research interests of individual faculty members. Tapes and individually supervised counseling sessions are employed to teach basic principles of parent counseling.

Finally, a comment should be made about the philosophy of using hospitalization for habilitation. Most of the usual discomforts of medical wards are ameliorated. After the initial evaluation, invasive medical procedures are rare, the children wear street clothes, and enforced boredom seldom occurs since the entire day is taken up by therapy programs. Any

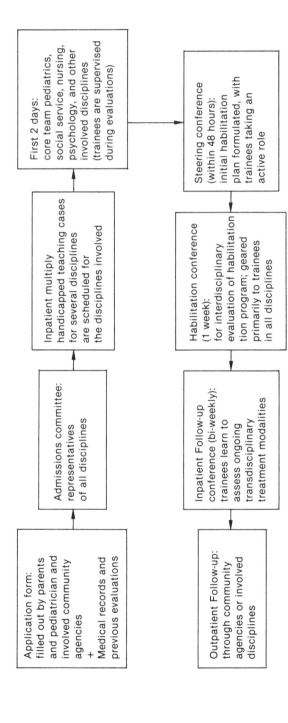

Figure 1. Flowchart for the inpatient rotation.

free time that remains is structured by an active child life program or an on-the-ward school for the older children. But the most positive aspect of inpatient habilitation is the ability to achieve rapid progress toward set developmental goals — children, parents, and therapists receive more than enough positive reinforcement from this visible improvement to outweigh the inconveniences of hospitalization.

Outpatient Services

Whereas the inpatient service focuses on the most severely involved multiply handicapped children in need of an intensive therapeutic regimen, the outpatient rotation, Child Development Clinic (CDC), involves the evaluation of patients with milder impairments, such as learning disabilities, borderline to mild mental retardation, and behavioral disorders. This division is somewhat artificial; the patients who have previously received evaluation and habilitation on the inpatient service continue to be followed in the outpatient clinic, and many outpatient children at some point in their follow-up develop problems best managed on the inpatient ward.

The outpatient flow process is similar to that for inpatients (see Figure 1), except that the time scale is somewhat extended. The pediatric fellow sees four new patients a week along with 8 to 12 follow-ups a week. Although a pediatric developmental assessment on a new patient takes approximately 3 hours, the initial complete evaluation takes 2 to 4 days. The steering conference and parent counseling session occurs 1 to 2 weeks afterward. To a slightly greater extent than on the inpatient service, the pediatric fellow will be able to follow his/her patient's evaluation through each of the disciplines. The steering conferences are organized as case-centered teaching sessions with senior faculty from each discipline in attendance. Specialized clinics, such as birth defects (meningomyelocele) and genetics, are part of this rotation, in addition to an afternoon a week at a community Health Maintenance Organization to provide developmental assessment services. A 2-year fellowship is necessary to give the pediatrician adequate time to follow up in the outpatient department the outcome of his/her recommendations for the patients he/she evaluates at the beginning of the fellowship. Failure to structure such an opportunity into the fellowship must be judged a serious flaw; there can be no "quickie" training programs in chronic handicapping conditions.

The outpatient fellow also sees all developmental consultation requests from the inpatient and outpatient services of the Johns Hopkins Hospital (most of these are from the Department of Pediatrics, with some from medicine and psychiatry, and they average about five per week). The fellow is individually supervised by a faculty member on his/her case formulation and recommendations. Many of these cases are referred for more comprehensive team evaluations and services.

While the CDC serves as the required outpatient rotation, there exists an elective rotation through the Diagnostic and Evaluation (D&E) clinic. The latter rotation sees the same types of patients and delivers very similar services. Apart from its source of funding, it differs little from the CDC except that it is more closely affiliated with other state and community agency health care delivery systems. In other university centers, such D&E clinics might easily serve as the principal outpatient teaching experience.

Pediatric Neurology Rotation

This experience enables the trainee to diagnose acute neurological complications of chronic disabilities and to rule out degenerative processes. During this 4-month period, the trainee participates in the evaluation and treatment of active neurological problems, such as head trauma, degenerative disorders, myopathies, neuropathies, and other acute neurological entities, as they are presented in an inpatient pediatric neurology service and the outpatient pediatric neurology clinics. The natural history and rehabilitation of severe head injuries and the management of complex seizure disorders (e.g., the West syndrome and the Lennox-Gastaut syndrome, both of which are frequently associated with mental retardation) are important aspects of pediatric neurology for the physician who wants to obtain special competence in the care of developmentally disabled children.

Child Psychiatry

The diagnosis and treatment of neurotic and psychotic disorders in the normal and the developmentally disabled population are studied. The pediatric trainee learns the techniques of management by both child psychiatrists and mental health counselors, and the dynamics of parent and sibling interactions are experienced within structured and supervised learning situations. This rotation is similar to a 1-month elective for pediatric residents, but its longer duration permits greater depth and the pediatric fellow's greater experience allows more primary responsibility.

Perinatology

The pediatric fellow follows the developmental progress of normal as well as high risk populations of full-term, premature, and small-for-date infants. He/she observes infant behavior along a temporal continuum from the newborn nursery into early childhood. The classic neonatology experience for pediatric residents focuses on acute medicine and life-and-death decisions. The pediatric fellow, on the other hand, makes developmental rounds in the intensive care nursery and follows the neurodevelopmental progress of infants during their stay in the nursery using such instruments as the Prechtl Examination, the Primitive Reflex Profile

(Capute et al., 1978), and the Brazelton Neonatal Behavior Scale. The fellow then continues to observe the development of the children in a service-oriented intensive care nursery follow-up clinic where a selected number of high risk infants receive primary health care while undergoing comprehensive developmental and biomedical evaluation. This conjoint effort with neonatology serves as both an ideal teaching clinic for the pediatric house staff as well as a fertile source of research data for neonatologists and developmentalists. In addition, a patient population can be identified that would not otherwise be receiving adequate well baby care. In university hospitals with such programs, this rotation should also be available to trainees in ambulatory pediatric fellowships.

EEG Laboratory

During the EEG laboratory rotation, the pediatric fellow becomes familiar with both the contributions and limitations of electroencephalography with regard to the management of children with chronic brain disorders. Auditory and visual evoked responses and other more experimental methodologies (such as brain stem responses) are studied. This rotation provides a useful substrate for the understanding and treatment of convulsive disorders in the handicapped population as well as an opportunity for doing clinical research.

Genetics and Biochemistry

The genetics and biochemistry rotation provides more formal exposure to clinical and laboratory genetics and to the various specialized techniques (amniocentesis, amino acid chromatography, and cytogenetics) in the biochemical evaluation of developmental disorders. It utilizes clinical material at both the Kennedy Institute and the Johns Hopkins Hospital and allows the trainee sufficient time and exposure to pursue research in these areas.

Other Training

A monthly journal club focuses on papers and journals not usually reviewed by pediatricians but of importance to the field of developmental disabilities. All fellows are required to present two prepared lectures a year on subjects of their choice before their peers. The developmental pediatrician, even if he/she does not pursue a formal academic career, will frequently be called upon to speak before community groups. Therefore, whatever other instructional benefit these lectures provide to the group, they are primarily intended as a source of constructive criticism in the mechanisms of communication for the neophyte speaker. Another important training experience is the appointment of each fellow to one of the hospital's committees (e.g., Medical Records, Utilization Review).

Distinctive Characteristics of the Program

The fellowship program has many distinctive characteristics. First, rather than focusing on a single entity, such as mental retardation or cerebral palsy, the program embraces the entire spectrum of developmental disabilities. Second, it employs a structured hierarchy of trainers with residents teaching medical students, fellows teaching residents, and faculty teaching fellows. This latter emphasis on introducing the importance of developmental phenomena throughout the medical school curriculum cannot be over-emphasized. It is very similar to the situation of ambulatory care: one cannot stress acute medicine from the first year of medical school to the last year of residency training and expect the finer points of ambulatory pediatrics to be magically absorbed in the process. Both developmental and ambulatory input need to be given more than lip service throughout medical training.[2]

OUTCOME

Forty-three fellows in developmental pediatrics have been trained at the John F. Kennedy Institute between July, 1965, and June, 1979. Of these fellows, 2 completed a 3-year program, while 32 completed a 2-year program. Of the nine fellows who completed only 1 year at the Institute, four received another year of formal training in developmental pediatrics at another University Affiliated Facility; of the five remaining, two completed child psychiatry residencies. Thus far the training program has produced two directors, one deputy director, and one coordinator of training at several University Affiliated Facilities. In addition, six of the graduates are actively involved in clinical research and one is involved in basic research. As an index of the program's impact on the pre-fellowship levels, of the 43 diplomates, 11 (26%) were former Johns Hopkins students and residents.[3]

The general pediatrician must be sensitive to the needs of the whole child — emotional as well as physical. The acquisition of this sensitivity is not currently subject to formal training, but is rather left to individual evaluation by program directors. The problem of influencing and measur-

---

[2]The important contributions that both these areas of pediatrics can and should make to one another within the context of fellowship training programs should be worked out within each individual university setting.

[3]Of the total group of 43 fellows, eight are currently involved in the private practice of developmental pediatrics (two of these have half-time academic appointments), nineteen are full-time academicians, seven work in D&E clinics, one is Director of Ambulatory Care at a university center, two are at the National Institute of Health, one directs a pediatric service at a U.S. naval hospital, one is employed at a state school, one is functioning as a geneticist, and another is employed in a private developmental center.

ing attitudinal responses is a particularly complex one in the area of developmental disabilities and we are far from any easy solution (see American Board of Pediatrics, Inc., 1974). Devising innovative techniques to develop and measure appropriate attitudinal responses on the part of trainees in both developmental and general pediatrics is one of the major tasks of the next decade. (Some preliminary approaches to this complex problem are discussed in various chapters of this book.)

CONCLUSION

The overall goal of this training program is to produce a pediatrician who possesses skills in coordinating and supervising the transdisciplinary and interdisciplinary evaluation and management of developmentally disabled children and their families. It is impossible for such post-doctoral fellowship training to exist in isolation. For effective implementation it must occur as a single facet in a comprehensive program in developmental pediatrics extending throughout the medical curriculum. With minor variations suited to individual training programs, the adoption of the model presented here should enhance the ability of most university centers to make significant contributions to reduce the substantial pediatric manpower shortage in the area of developmental disabilities (see The Task Force on Pediatric Education, 1978).

REFERENCES

Accardo, P. J., and Capute, A. J. 1979. The pediatrician and the developmentally delayed child. Monographs in Developmental Pediatrics, Vol. II. Baltimore: University Park Press.

American Board of Pediatrics, Inc., 1974. Foundations for Evaluating the Competency of Pediatricians. Chicago: American Board of Pediatrics, Inc.

Capute, A. J., Accardo, P. J., Vining, E. P. G., Rubenstein, J., and Harryman, S. 1978. Primitive reflex profile. Monographs in Developmental Pediatrics, Vol. I. Baltimore: University Park Press.

The Task Force on Pediatric Education. 1978. The future of pediatric education. Evanston, Ill.: American Academy of Pediatrics.

chapter 13

CONTINUING EDUCATION OF PHYSICIANS IN DEVELOPMENTAL DIAGNOSIS

William K. Frankenburg and Marlin E. Cohrs

Fifteen years ago our research team began work in the area of developmental screening in an effort to design procedures that would promote the early identification of handicapped children in a cost-efficient manner (Frankenburg, 1967). At that time we wanted to advance screening and identification methods and to demonstrate the need for more diagnostic services and facilities for developmentally handicapped children. During the ensuing years we have developed procedures that have been utilized internationally to screen hundreds of thousands of children annually (Frankenburg and Dodds, 1967). At that time we wanted to advance screening and identification methods and to demonstrate the need for more diagnostic services and facilities for developmentally handicapped children. During the ensuing years we have developed procedures that have been utilized internationally to screen hundreds of thousands of children annually (Frankenburg, Goldstein, and Camp, 1971; Frankenburg et al., 1976). Such large scale acceptance of screening has, in part, been the result of increased public awareness of the importance of early identification of children with handicaps. This awareness has been translated into numerous federal programs, such as Child Find and Early Periodic Screening, Diagnosis, and Treatment, and has been evidenced by the recommendations of governmental agencies and professional organizations like the American Academy of Pediatrics. Such recommendations call for routine screening to identify, as early as possible, any child in need of diagnosis and treatment.

About four years ago we turned our attention to the goal of developing better diagnostic services for handicapped children since there is an urgent need for such expanded and improved services. The evaluation of developmentally suspect children by multidisciplinary teams has, in the United States, been the recommended method for diagnostic appraisal. Indeed, the value of such a team approach cannot be denied; however, there are certain drawbacks to confining ourselves exclusively to its use.

Multidisciplinary team evaluations, which are quite expensive and time-consuming, are not readily available to children in all communities, and there are simply not enough centers offering this type of evaluation to meet the expected needs of the population. If all of the currently mandated and recommended screening programs were to be implemented, virtually every child in this country would undergo developmental screening several times before reaching 6 years of age. A conservative estimate is that 10% of the children being screened require diagnostic evaluation and periodic reevaluation. Thus, it becomes clear that existing diagnostic facilities are gravely inadequate. It is, therefore, of the utmost urgency that massive nationwide efforts be undertaken to train professionals in diagnostic evaluation.

THE PHYSICIAN TRAINING PROGRAM: RATIONALE

Having evaluated children, both as part of a team and individually, we have come to the conclusion that not every child who is suspect on screening or whose parents are concerned about the child's developmental status needs a complete multidisciplinary evaluation. Instead, about 80% of the children who are suspect on screening can be satisfactorily evaluated by family practitioners and pediatricians who have been specially trained in diagnostic testing. Those children who have very complex psychosocial problems or who are severely multiply handicapped would require a more exhaustive evaluation by a multidisciplinary diagnostic team.

On the basis of this assumption, we feel that it would be possible to train both primary care physicians who are in residency training, as well as those physicians who are in actual practice, to consider the differential diagnosis of developmental problems and to perform the necessary basic diagnostic evaluations. In this respect, we perceive four functions of the primary care physician:

1. To make a categorical diagnosis and thereby establish the cause for the problem by:
   a. Identifying medical problems, such as neurological disorders and muscular, metabolic, and genetic diseases.
   b. Identifying sensory disorders, such as ophthalmological and auditory problems, that contribute to the cause of the child's de-

velopmental problems or that may, if not identified and cor-
rected, limit the efficacy of intervention programs.

  c. Identifying socioemotional disorders, such as deprivation, aber-
rant parenting, and psychiatric disorders, that would require immediate treatment.

  d. Identifying speech and language disorders that would require
treatment.

  e. Identifying the child's level of functioning and thereby determining if there is a significant delay.

2. To determine whether or not the child should be referred for further
evaluation either by physicians or allied health workers, such as oph-
thalmologists, psychiatrists, neurologists, geneticists, endocrinolo-
gists, physical and occupational therapists, speech pathologists, and
educators.

3. To assemble the diverse test results into a comprehensive and coherent plan. This function actually might be performed through an interdisciplinary staffing.

4. To counsel families on the meaning of the evaluation findings, answer their questions, and map out a plan of action to help the child
and his/her family.

Some physicians may carry out each of these four functions. Others
may choose to work as part of a team and, in that capacity, limit themselves to identifying medical problems. In this case, others in the community will determine which allied health consultants will be asked to
evaluate the child. Generally, the role of the physician will depend upon
his/her own inclinations and the local community patterns for serving
handicapped children.

FORMAT OF INSTRUCTION

As stated previously, as many as 10% of the nation's children may require
annual diagnostic evaluation. If so, it may be assumed that at least one-
half of the nation's pediatricians and family practitioners will require
training in developmental diagnosis, since few physicians have previously
acquired the necessary skills in this area. Therefore, our broad goal has
been to develop a concise, economical program that would lend itself to
nationwide replication. To assure that the replicated program is similar to
the original in scope and content requires careful packaging of the training materials. Since no one has previously developed a protocol for developmental diagnosis, we felt that any protocol that we might develop
would have to lend itself to periodic revision. Furthermore, the lessons
would have to be presented in a flexible format so as to allow their use in
varying circumstances in different parts of the country.

With these conditions set forth, it was decided to utilize both videotape and print media. Videotape, which lends itself to immediate review and modification at a relatively low cost, was chosen as the primary method of delivery and has proven very effective for demonstrating techniques and procedures. Printed outlines and summaries, which are economical to produce, copy, and distribute, are provided to reinforce the video presentation and to serve as tools for further reference. Although black and white television equipment is far less expensive than color and is as effective in teaching as color, we elected to utilize color equipment because it shows the nature of skin lesions and other conditions better and has greater student viewing appeal.

In selecting the video medium for teaching, we recognized a number of serious drawbacks to television teaching. These limitations are:

1. Television does not stop to answer questions.
2. It does not allow time for group discussion.
3. It is inefficient for conducting drill.
4. It does not adjust to individual student differences.
5. It encourages a passive form of learning, which does not always promote retention of knowledge.

In spite of these drawbacks, we felt that video had much to offer and considered what made educational television programs, such as Sesame Street, Chicago City TV College, Australian School of the Year, and Bavarian Telecollege, so effective. In general these programs may be characterized by the following:

1. The programs were designed for specific audiences.
2. They had clearly defined educational objectives that were relevant to the audience.
3. They used technology that was most effective in presenting the proposed content.
4. They used instructors who were trained beforehand, who were knowledgeable in the subject being taught, and who presented the materials in a well-organized manner.
5. The instructors were charismatic and were interested in the use of the TV medium.
6. They used other media to promote interaction between audience members.
7. They evaluated the educational effectiveness and modified the materials to enhance the effectiveness of the lessons.

We have attempted to utilize these positive aspects of program design in the preparation of the Physicians Training Program. In addition, the approach we have selected was considerably influenced by the work of

Gibbons, Kincheloe, and Down (1977) who developed a technique called "tutored videotape instruction" for off-campus graduate engineering students of Stanford University. In essence, their technique was to videotape unrehearsed, unedited lessons from classroom courses and to show them to small groups of 3 to 10 students who were assisted by paraprofessional tutors. This technique was based on the premise that students learn more from a lecture when they feel free to interrupt and ask for explanation of a point or concept. This project demonstrated that students learned best when the videotapes were interrupted every 5 to 10 minutes for 3 to 5 minutes of group discussion. The technique was less effective for use with only one or two students and for very large groups. Thus, their technique combined the best elements of a lecture — that is to say, depth and continuity of subject matter — with the best elements of small group discussions to assure that the lecturers respond to individual needs and differences.

Our approach, which is still evolving, has involved the preparation of a training outline to describe all of the lessons in the program. Each lesson is developed in the following manner:

1. A protocol is designed to specify what the physician is to do.
2. Lesson goals and objectives are defined.
3. An outline of the lesson is developed.
4. A script is written for the lesson.
5. Project staff review the scripts.
6. The lesson is revised.
7. The lessons are edited by a professional editor.
8. A "story board" with visual aids for the TV presentation is developed.
9. The author rehearses the script for the TV presentation.
10. The lesson is videotaped by a staff member using a portable color video camera.
11. The lesson undergoes immediate internal review and is modified and retaped when necessary.
12. The lesson instructor develops a bibliography, examination questions and answers, and suggested times for interrupting the lessons, as well as a list of topics for discussion. (These materials are used by the tutors to guide student learning.)
13. Copies of the lessons are printed for student use.
14. Both the written script and the videotaped lesson undergo external evaluation.
    a. The written text is sent to three national experts in the specific field for critique.
    b. The videotaped lesson is evaluated by the students (in terms of the manner of the presentation, duration, relevance) and by the

Table 1.   Course outline

I.	*Identification of Developmentally Delayed Children*	
	Chapter 1	Introduction to Screening
	Chapter 2	Rationale for Early Identification and Treatment
	Chapter 3	Developmental Screening
II.	*Diagnosis of Developmentally Delayed Children*	
	Chapter 4	Introduction to Diagnostic Evaluation
	Chapter 5	Medical History and Physical Examination
	Chapter 6	Neurological Evaluation
	Chapter 7	Neuromotor Evaluation
	Chapter 8	Genetic Evaluation
	Chapter 9	Metabolic Evaluation
	Chapter 10	Ophthalmological Evaluation
	Chapter 11	Audiological Evaluation
	Chapter 12	Speech and Language Evaluation
	Chapter 13	Psychiatric Evaluation
	Chapter 14	Psychological Evaluation
	Chapter 15	Environmental Evaluation
III.	*Comprehensive Approach to Follow-Up*	
	Chapter 16	Educational Planning
	Chapter 17	Public Health Nursing Referral
	Chapter 18	The Case Review
	Chapter 19	Parent Counseling

tutors (in terms of the lesson content and materials, topics discussed, questions raised, and suggested changes in the lesson). Classroom instruction is further evaluated by examining the students' acquisition of knowledge, as evidenced by their performance on the final test, and by studying recommendations of project staff who have observed the classroom instruction.

On the basis of these evaluations, some lessons have been deleted, others have been modified, and most have been totally rewritten and retaped. The current training program includes: the semi-tutorial classroom instruction designed for 8 to 15 students at one time, a period during which students can practice what they have learned, and time for individual case review.

The classroom instruction takes 20 hours and is divided into three parts (see Table 1). The first part, a discussion of screening, attempts to motivate physicians to undertake developmental screening so as to identify children requiring a diagnostic evaluation. This part consists of three chapters and takes approximately two hours for viewing and discussion.

The second part, which focuses on diagnosis, is designed to teach the physician a protocol or an algorithm to be followed in the evaluation of children who are suspect of having a developmental problem. This part consists of 12 chapters and takes 16 hours of classroom instruction.

The final segment of the physician's training program, four chapters requiring approximately 2 hours, is designed to teach primary care physicians how to plan and implement the most effective treatment for developmentally delayed children. Included in this portion of the program are descriptions of educational planning and public health nursing referrals. In addition, lessons are designed to teach physicians how to pull together the diverse findings of experts from many disciplines into a comprehensive treatment plan and how to impart diagnostic treatment information to parents of a handicapped child. Finally, this segment includes information relating to techniques for improving sensitivity to the affective responses of parents so that intervention and treatment will be most effective.

In addition to the video cassette, each lesson includes a printed outline and videoscript that emphasizes the importance of identifying the problem under discussion, a protocol for identifying the problem, recommendations of when, where, and how to refer for consultation, and indications for laboratory procedures. For each lesson there is a bibliography of additional reading, a set of examination questions, and a form for the student's evaluation of the lesson. The tutor's guide consists of suggested topics for discussion during that lesson, relevant reprints or articles, answers to student examination questions, and a form for the tutor's evaluation of the lesson.

Further revisions of the training materials will be made on the basis of the above evaluations and on the basis of additional evaluations, which will be conducted at the time of case review. If the results show that students failed to follow the path of our algorithm, we must determine whether we should modify the instruction. While this is a process evaluation, we think that it is very important.

NATIONAL FIELD TESTING

We shall make the entire training program available to five University Affiliated Facilities (UAFs) for field testing. Further revisions will be made and an additional field test with other UAFs will also be conducted. After that we shall develop a "quasi-final product." Originally we had planned to develop a final version and to videotape it in a professional studio. However, we have instead decided to abandon this idea because we consider our "home-developed videotapes" to be of reasonably good quality and because we do not want the program to be considered as either the final word or the one-and-only approach to developmental diagnosis. As other points of view become apparent and new knowledge becomes available, further revisions, which will be made by others and by ourselves, can be easily inserted into the program.

ORGANIZATION OF THE TRAINING PROGRAM

Our training program is jointly sponsored by the John F. Kennedy (JFK) Child Development Center, which is a University Affiliated Facility and an integral part of the University of Colorado Medical Center; the Colorado Chapter of the American Academy of Pediatrics; the University of Colorado Medical Center's Division of Continuing Education; the Colorado State Departments of Education and Health; and the national Office of Developmental Disabilities. The Colorado Chapter of the American Academy of Pediatrics has informed all of its Colorado members about our training program, and the JFK Center has informed family physicians in Colorado, as well as pediatricians in Wyoming, about the program. Physicians who are interested in participating notify the JFK Center by a postcard that was included in the informational material. The JFK Center then collates all requests on a regional basis. When 5 to 10 physicians in a region request such training, the chairman of the Continuing Education Committee of the Colorado Chapter of the American Academy of Pediatrics contacts the appropriate regional representative regarding the names of the interested pediatricians. The representative then contacts them and other local pediatricians and family practitioners to tell them that training in developmental diagnosis is being scheduled in their locale. In this way, additional names of physicians desiring to take such training are accumulated. The representative also selects a time for the training (it may be scheduled on weekends or during the week) and makes the necessary local arrangements for the training.

In the meantime, the JFK Center finds a tutor, who is usually one of the former graduates of the Center's 1-year training program in developmental diagnosis. Most of these tutors are involved in private practice and sometimes reside in the region where the training will take place. Although these physicians are too busy to devote time to developing a training program, they are extremely pleased to conduct such training for a number of reasons: 1) it provides them with an updated review of developmental diagnosis, 2) they enjoy teaching and assisting their local colleagues, and 3) the training makes them visible to their colleagues and perhaps will generate a few referrals. The students can readily identify with these tutors because they, too, are engaged in general pediatric practice. In addition, class discussions reveal many similarities between the practices of the role-modeling tutors and their students.

The University's Division of Continuing Education offers 24 hours of CM-1 credit to all graduates of the program. The American Academy of Family Practice gives a similar number of credits. This number is half the number required for Colorado relicensure and half that required to remain in good standing with the Academy of Family Practice.

The State Department of Education receives the names of physicians who have completed this training so they can refer children to these physicians for the necessary evaluations as set forth by Public Law 94-142. The State Health Department refers to the training project those physicians working in its Developmental and Evaluation Clinics when they request such training. In addition, attempts are made to coordinate referral and diagnostic evaluations between the private physicians and the State Developmental and Evaluation Clinics.

The federal Office of Developmental Disabilities, which has funded the production of this training program, bears the cost of preparing the lessons, which includes the Center project staff, the AV equipment, the videotapes, and related expenses. Student tuition pays the cost of conducting the training in various parts of the state. In the past, we have charged practicing physicians $75 to cover the cost of their $10 syllabus and the cost of the tutor, who is paid at the rate of $100 per day. Physicians who are in residency training either in family practice or in pediatrics pay only the $10 fee for the syllabus. These fees will have to be increased slightly in order to cover some of the unanticipated costs such as videotape wear and tear, TV tapedeck maintenance and replacement, and increased printing costs. Despite the anticipated increase to $100 for practitioners and $12.50 for residents, the cost per CM-1 credit will only be $4 per hour as opposed to the usual $5 per hour. For this sum, the students receive semi-tutorial instruction and an extensive syllabus.

One anticipated benefit of this program is that it will begin to bridge the costly gap between health providers and educators. By observing the training program, the local directors of special education and developmental disabilities can see the essential components in the diagnostic evaluation. They can learn to appreciate the value of such an evaluation and to answer questions regarding therapeutic and educational programs. In this way, a smooth flow of referrals should be facilitated.

Currently, the total number of physicians trained through this program as of May 1979 is 99. We have received requests for training from many more phyicians but are at this time reluctant to enroll too many trainees at once since the lessons are still being revised.

SUMMARY

This chapter has described a unique attempt at providing short-term training in developmental diagnosis for residents and practitioners of pediatrics and family practice. The training program's unusual elements are:

1. The program offers semi-tutorial instruction by a tutor who utilizes previously prepared videotapes and printed materials.

2. Each lesson consists of the printed lesson, outline of the lesson, bibliography, examination questions and answers, and a tutor's lesson guide.

3. The program has very high appeal to the students who see it as a way of filling a gap in their training, learning to provide more comprehensive service to their patients, and earning continuing education credits. The program is also seen as being relevant to their practices, useful, responsive to their individual concerns, and provided in a very convenient manner.

4. The program is highly flexible in the hours and location of training, as well as in the content. Adjustments for local circumstances can be made by changing the printed instructions, such as when and where to make referrals and where to send the laboratory specimens. Furthermore, the sequence of lessons can be altered easily since no lesson is dependent on another, and tutors can elect to delete a lesson and to add or replace a lesson by developing their own. Similarly, lessons can be updated with little effort.

5. Last, but not least, after the lessons have been developed, the training pays for itself through the modest tuition charge.

We do not see this program as the answer to all of the diagnostic problems. Instead, it is an initial effort that undoubtedly will undergo many changes during the next few years. We hope that the program will entice others to develop alternative approaches to meet the diagnostic needs of this nation's handicapped children.

REFERENCES

Frankenburg, W. K., and Dodds, J. B. 1967. The Denver Developmental Screening Test. The Journal of Pediatrics, 71, 181-191.
Frankenburg, W. K., Goldstein, A. D., and Camp, B. W. 1971. The revised Denver Developmental Screening Test: Its accuracy as a screening instrument. The Journal of Pediatrics, 79, 988-995.
Frankenburg, W. K., van Doorninck, W. J., Liddell, T. N., and Dick, N. P. 1976. The Denver Prescreening Developmental Questionnaire (PDQ). Pediatrics, 57, 744-753.
Gibbons, J. F., Kincheloe, W. R., and Down, K. S. 1977. Tutored videotaped instruction: Use of electronics media in education. Science, 195 (4283), 1139-1146.

chapter 14
CONTINUING EDUCATION OF PEDIATRICIANS ON THE NEEDS OF THE EXCEPTIONAL CHILD

Peter W. Zinkus and Marvin I. Gottlieb

The traditional role of the general pediatrician has sustained increasing change in recent years. With more of the life-threatening diseases of childhood coming under adequate control, the pediatrician has increasingly been called upon to focus his/her attention on the problems of the exceptional child. As the first professional likely to see the child and follow developmental progress during the first several years of life, the pediatrician is in a unique position to provide early detection, diagnosis, and treatment for the exceptional child. It is recognized that many subtle yet chronic handicapping conditions, such as learning disabilities, speech and language delays, and other developmental disorders, which can reduce the quality of life for the child in future years, can be detected early, thereby offering a more optimistic prognosis. In most cases, the pediatrician stands as the first line of defense in effecting the early and critical therapeutic measures. Until recently, however, only a handful of programs offered the physician-in-training the necessary exposure to the management of the exceptional child.

The importance of continuing education for pediatricians on the needs of the exceptional child has been reinforced by recent plans for the recertification of practicing physicians. Proposals by the American Academy of Pediatrics (AAP) (1976) define the recertification program as "closely tied to a program of continuing education emphasizing both recent advances in comprehensive (general) pediatrics and areas of specialized interest within pediatrics." The recertification program includes reviews of twelve major categories of pediatric practice. The categories that are significant to the needs of the exceptional child are the areas of continuing education involving:

1. Handicapped children
2. Chronic illness, death, and dying
3. Growth and development
4. Behavioral pediatrics
5. Emotional and psychosocial problems
6. Family dynamics and counseling
7. Mental retardation
8. Learning disabilities
9. School adjustment problems
10. Adolescent medicine
11. Delinquency and drug abuse

Accordingly, recognition of the role of the pediatrician in the detection, the diagnosis, and the management of the exceptional child appears to have become a reality. Continuing education appears to be the strategy of choice to improve health care delivery by meeting the needs of the exceptional child on the primary care level.

The American Academy of Pediatrics (Charney, 1976) has also addressed the future role of the general pediatrician as a primary health care provider. One such role of the pediatrician includes that of an "advocate" for the exceptional child (Kenny and Clemmens, 1975). As an advocate, the general pediatrician's need to familiarize and improve his/her competence in dealing with such areas as school health, developmental retardation, behavioral problems, cerebral palsy, and other chronic handicapping conditions is stressed.

Continuing education of the practicing pediatrician becomes even more significant in light of this changing role for the general pediatrician. Many communities are not in close proximity to large medical centers with their abundance of specialists and expertise in dealing with the exceptional child. Many times the pediatrician must serve as the child advocate in coordinating a multidisciplinary evaluation and effecting a therapeutic program. Therefore, in addition to the role in early detection and diagnosis of the exceptional child, the pediatrician's role as coordinator and advocate becomes highly significant.

THE ONE-WEEK INTENSIVE STUDY PROGRAM

At the University of Tennessee Center for the Health Sciences, Section of Developmental and Behavioral Pediatrics of the Department of Pediatrics, practicing pediatricians gain expertise in dealing with the problems of the exceptional child through clinical and didactic exposure as well as through outreach programs. Intensive training is aimed at meeting the needs of the pediatrician-in-practice in a practical and useful yet comprehensive manner.

One approach involves didactic and clinical exposure on the university campus during which practicing physicians spend 3 to 5 days in intensive study on the needs of the exceptional child. During this time, didactic approaches are utilized to familiarize physicians with the basic terminology and issues related to the exceptional child. Lectures are combined with audiovisual techniques, discussion, and opportunities for additional self-study. Lecture topics are directed toward the problems most commonly encountered by a practicing physician with the exceptional child. The physician is familiarized with several sides of controversial issues (e.g., minimal brain dysfunction, hyperactivity) rather than receiving a unilateral theoretical approach. Major lecture topics emphasize the relative meaning of the term *exceptional* from a medical perspective, placing exceptionality in a medical framework with analyses of definitions, etiology, incidence, classification, signs and symptoms, therapies, and prognoses. In addition, instruction is provided on the role of the physician in managing the exceptional child, differential diagnosis, interdisciplinary evaluations, and case history reviews.

In the clinical setting, practicing pediatricians participate in an established clinic for exceptional children for periods up to 1 week and are exposed to a variety of chronic handicapping conditions of childhood such as problems in delayed speech, learning disabilities, mental retardation, or neurological disorders. Major emphasis is placed upon early diagnosis and therapeutic programming as part of the physician's responsibility. In addition, through working contact with a multidisciplinary team, the physician is made aware of the techniques for coordinating professional efforts in a number of disciplines and translating the results into meaningful therapeutic endeavors.

THE MINI-RESIDENCY

In the near future, the Department of Academic Affairs and Continuing Education will institute a "Mini-Residency" program incorporating many of the concepts of effective treatment of the exceptional child into an intensive 1- to 2-week course for practicing physicians. This program will include the many critical knowledge and skill areas needed by physicians for competent management of the exceptional child. The proposed program will offer the practicing physician:

1. Contact with the spectrum of exceptional children and their problems.

2. The opportunity to work in close contact with a multidisciplinary team, including psychologists, social workers, speech and language therapists, special educators, nurse practitioners, child development specialists, and other professionals. The physician will gain an appreciation of the contribution of each discipline and an awareness of the need for coordination of the therapeutic program based upon their evaluations.

3. Techniques in the examination of the exceptional child. In addition to the usual physical examination, special neurological techniques, as well as methods for screening for problems in perceptual and academic areas, will be taught.

4. Field trips to community agencies. These trips will be conducted to gain an appreciation of the methods of assessment and referral as well as to monitor a child's progress.

5. Management of the exceptional child in private practice. Often the physician must perform basic evaluations in a private practice setting. Numerous evaluation instruments have been devised to assess the developmental, emotional, and educational status of a high risk or delayed child. Many instruments can be administered by office personnel and scored easily and quickly by computer services. With the high costs involved in multidisciplinary evaluations, the physician can learn to select further evaluations based upon his/her own examination in combination with easily administered scales. Management in the private office setting requires attention to thorough and complete diagnostic intervention with additional emphasis on minimizing cost to the family. These factors are recognized and will be included in the mini-residency teaching program.

OUTREACH PROGRAMS

Many individuals cannot take 1 or 2 weeks away from a busy practice to participate in the intensive, on-campus activities. Recognizing this limitation, programs of intensive education of shorter duration have been developed. These outreach activities are included in the continuing education program for physicians on the needs of the exceptional child.

One major activity is the Leigh Buring Conference on the Exceptional Child,[1] which is convened once a year to provide a 2-day exposure to the exceptional child, family, and community. The format includes lectures and workshops covering a variety of topics such as the office man-

---

[1] This conference is approved for credit by the American Academy of Family Physicians and the American Medical Association.

agement of the exceptional child. These workshops serve as a model for physicians to use in their own practice. The most recent conference included such topics as: the neurological basis for learning and behavior, the child with speech and communicative disorders, reading disabilities, diagnosis of visual and auditory perceptual deficits, management of the hyperkinetic child through various modalities of treatment, the learning disabled juvenile delinquent as a case for early intervention in learning disabilities, and techniques of audiological, speech, and language intervention.

Finally, additional outreach programs are offered through participation in area medical meetings. Lectures and discussions, as well as workshops, on the exceptional child are offered. Techniques of detection, diagnosis, and treatment are discussed and complemented by access to evaluation materials and self-study references.

SUMMARY

The changing role of the general pediatrician is becoming oriented more toward the needs of the exceptional child. Walzer and Richmond (1973) pointed out this change in emphasis when they noted:

> As the life threatening disorders have become less of a major problem in child health, the attention of the biomedical sciences has gradually shifted to more subtle problems. We are now focusing our investigations on the prevention and treatment of those handicapping disorders which — although not life threatening — do result in a serious loss of human potential (p. 549).

Continuing education for the practicing physician in this area is a necessary but complex undertaking. The needs of the exceptional child require competent and effective medical management, and, for some physicians, a significant investment in the study of new methods and techniques is essential. The nature of the subject matter includes a wide range of organic, psycho-social, and educational factors, all of which contribute in varying degrees to the difficulties of the exceptional child. Appreciation of these complexities is the first step in effective treatment. In this sense, familiarity with the needs of the exceptional child may succeed in removing the term exceptional from the medical vocabulary. The physician, armed with knowledge and confidence, need not view a developmentally disabled or learning impaired child as any more exceptional than the child with a common infectious disease. Although we attempt to train medical students and residents in this basic philosophy, continuing education provides improved health care for the exceptional child by making such care an integral part of the pediatrician's challenge.

REFERENCES

American Academy of Pediatrics. 1976. Recertification plan. News and Comment, 27, 2–3.

Charney, E. 1976. The general pediatrician and the future of primary care. News and Comment, 27, 10–11.

Kenny, T. J., and Clemmens, R. L. 1975. Behavioral Pediatrics and Child Development. Baltimore: Williams & Wilkins Company.

Walzer, S., and Richmond, B. R. 1973. The epidemiology of learning disorders, The Pediatric Clinics of North America, 20, 549–565.

chapter 15
PEDIATRIC NEUROLOGY AND THE MANAGEMENT OF DEVELOPMENTAL DISABILITIES

Gerhard E. Martin

For a number of years, certain medical disciplines, such as family medicine, psychiatry, and pediatrics, have been at the center of public discussion and even public criticism with regard to their clinical practice and general health care responsibilities for exceptional children and their families. Although no such attention has been focused on either neurology in general or on pediatric neurology in particular, the implementation of Public Law 94-142, the Education for All Handicapped Children Act of 1975, will undoubtedly expand the participation of these disciplines, including pediatric neurology, in the evaluation, diagnosis, and management of children with chronic developmental problems. It is the purpose of this chapter to outline a rationale for the involvement of pediatric neurologists, to describe their role as part of the diagnostic and treatment process, and to present implications for training. In general, the chapter focuses attention on the role of the pediatric neurologist in the management of developmental disabilities.

From a developmental perspective, neurological integrity is clearly one prerequisite for optimal cognitive and psychosocial development. In order for impairments of this integrity to be considered in the context of children's developmental and experiential needs, they must be identified and functionally defined as accurately as possible. This calls for a highly detailed and comprehensive evaluation of the developmental potentials of such children, the careful and sophisticated formulation of a multidimensional prognosis, a problem-oriented approach to long-term manage-

ment, and last but not least, an increase in communication and cooperation with other child care professionals, many of them nonmedical, as
well as parents.

INVOLVEMENT OF THE PEDIATRIC NEUROLOGIST

The anticipated increased need for the involvement of pediatric neurologists with handicapped children will have to be reconciled with other demands on the neurologist's time. These include clinical management of
acute, as opposed to chronic, neurological disorders, teaching, research,
and the reality of limited manpower. In the area of pediatric neurology,
the Joint Commission on Neurology of the American Neurological Association (Yahr, 1975), adopting parts of a 1970 study by the National Institute of Neurological Diseases and Stroke, projected a need for one pediatric neurologist engaged in patient care for a population of every 100,000
children, in addition to 170 academic pediatric neurological teams at a
ratio of 3 pediatric neurologists per team. Following the establishment of
a new certificate by the American Board of Psychiatry and Neurology in
1968 qualifying the diplomate as a neurologist with special competence in
child neurology, the number of board certified pediatric neurologists is
now somewhat short of 250. Considering both a future increase in the
pediatric neurological manpower as well as a predicted child population
of over 63 million under the age of 18 by 1980 (The Task Force on Pediatric Education, 1978), the number of qualified pediatric neurologists in the
near future will meet only 30%-50% of the projected need. To compound
matters further, the Joint Commission has estimated that approximately
one-third of all neurologists spend full time in research, education, administration, or federal services, and that even among the remainder,
only slightly more than half of their time is devoted to direct patient care
activities.

Thus, for pediatric neurologists to be able to provide and/or secure
support for neurologically handicapped children, their parents, and the
interdisciplinary habilitation teams in an effective manner, very comprehensive, efficient, and personal *consultation* skills will have to be developed. Furthermore, it appears essential that pediatric neurologists become more cognizant of the complex developmental, social, emotional,
and educational implications and functional dynamics operative in such
children and their families, as well as the diagnostic and habilitation skills
of other child care professionals. In addition, they must become comfortable in assisting with the identification and ordering of sequential priorities of intervention within an interdisciplinary model.

Commitment to the Management of Developmental Disabilities

The necessity for pediatric neurologists to become actively involved in the complex and interdisciplinary habilitation process of handicapped children has been recognized, and some of the appropriate logistics have been defined and detailed in countries such as Sweden and Great Britain (Hagbert, Ingram, and MacKeith, 1970). In the United States, leaders in pediatric neurology have expressed a strong commitment to the care of these children (Carter, 1971). For example, Swaiman (1974), in a major address, stated that:

> The developing nervous system with which we deal determines the individual's social, occupational and behavioral adjustment to life...children who suffer from cerebral palsy, epilepsy, learning disabilities, organic behavior disorders, and mental retardation — all suffer from afflictions of the nervous system that require our expertise...if we are not prepared to train physicians to manage these neurological problems and to take part in their direct care, others will fill the vacuum...only if we train future pediatric neurologists to meet the broad needs of the children to whom we are committed shall we justify the perpetuation of our specialty (p. 809).

However, a review of standard textbooks in pediatric neurology reveals that the overwhelming portion of these texts is devoted to etiology, pathology, diagnosis, and inpatient treatment. Sequelae to acute neurological conditions are, as a rule, treated as unfortunate and unalterable chronic outcomes rather than as dynamic deficits that, in the developing child, will become compounded by environmental factors when not managed properly. There is usually no more than a passing reference to the potentially devastating effects of the interaction between neurological and environmental factors, the need for problem- and habilitation-oriented long-term management of chronic, nonprogressive neurological disabilities, and the logistics of the necessary interdisciplinary interaction and cooperation. Clearly we must focus more attention on the fact that these deficits can be modified, ameliorated, compensated for, and, at times, overcome.

Further support for the fact that management of developmental disabilities has received insufficient attention can be found by examining the questions in Volume 35 of the *Medical Examination Review Book* (Bresnan, Nakano, and Snodgrass, 1978). Chronic developmental disabilities (excluding seizure disorders) are dealt with in about 7% out of a total of 2,000 questions. However, only a fraction of these questions are concerned with the strategies of long-term management.

Current Activities of the Practitioner   But then, how realistic are these concerns? How do they relate to the day-to-day practice of a pediatric neurologist? Do they reflect concrete needs or are they merely representative of a public criticism of the health care delivery system and a vaguely defined demand to make it "more efficient and humane, and better able to provide adequate health care to all those in need" (Earnest, 1978, p. 2).

The truth of the matter is that we do not really know at this time what pediatric neurologists do. There has been no carefully conducted representative survey similar to that carried out in pediatrics (The Task Force on Pediatric Education, 1978). Therefore, relevant evidence must come from an examination of existing individual reports and a review of clinical data.

In Canada, Tibbles (1976) reviewed a total of 2,018 consecutive office referrals to one pediatric neurologist serving a well-delineated geographical area in the eastern part of the country with a population of approximately one million. Excluding seizure disorders (24%) and metabolic diseases (0.8%), 30% of the referrals were for such chronically handicapping conditions as cerebral palsy, prenatal malformations, speech and language problems, auditory or visual impairments, behavior problems, childhood autism, and unqualified mental retardation (13%). Unfortunately, the author did not indicate how frequently a chronic neurological handicap existed or developed in conditions such as complex partial seizures, infectious diseases, trauma, and vascular disorders.

Weichsel (1974) analyzed the first one hundred pediatric neurological consultations in a community hospital setting in Lansing, Michigan. In this study, 25% of the children were diagnosed as being mentally retarded, with 10% more evidencing other chronic developmental disabilities such as arrested hydrocephalus, undiagnosed CNS anomaly, multiple congenital anomalies, tuberous sclerosis, and neurologically impaired status after head trauma or encephalitis. Similar to the Tibbles report, an additional 21% of the children were afflicted with chronic convulsive disorders. In these latter disorders, the frequency of adverse social and educational implications has led to their recognition as a developmental disability in this country.

Accordingly, from these reports, on a day-to-day basis the practitioner does appear to be faced with significant management problems of a chronic nature. In addition, in view of the implied habilitation needs and potential of the younger children, it is important to note that one-third of the referred children were under 3 years of age.

DOMAINS OF THE PEDIATRIC NEUROLOGIST

Placing training, manpower, and management concerns aside for the moment, let us look at some of the areas of manifest or potential chronic neurological handicap where the pediatric neurologist can be most helpful, and most productive. For simplicity of presentation, these handicaps are organized and discussed in terms of major disability categories.

Minimal Brain Dysfunction

Carter (1971) has placed particular emphasis upon the professional involvement of pediatric neurologists with children suffering from learning disabilities (LD) or minimal brain dysfunction (MBD). The incidence of MBD in this country is estimated to be 5%–15% in the general population and as high as 28% in underprivileged children (Eisenberg, 1966). With regard to the child's clinical manifestations in the educational setting, the syndrome is often viewed as a nosological entity. In reality, however, the etiology is quite heterogeneous and often multifactorial (Wender, 1971). There is a spectrum from those children where primary and presumed developmental dyslexia or hyperactivity is organically based (Bergström and Bille, 1978), to those where both problems develop subsequent to a variety of adverse environmental factors (Pearson, 1952). The majority of the children seem to be somewhere along this continuum. The so-called soft neurological signs, frequently mentioned in the literature, may be just one expression of a true perceptual or integrational cerebral deficit, or they may represent no more than a concomitant to minimal to mild motor handicap with no cause and effect relation to the child's reading or other learning difficulties whatsoever. However, eventually most of these children will find themselves trapped in a vicious cycle due to their primary weaknesses. What often follows are adverse parental reactions and secondary failure in other areas such as scholastic performance. This, in turn, often leads to the frequent occurrence of behavior problems.

Due to the correlation with soft neurological signs and often abnormal EEGs (Capute, Niedermeyer, and Richardson, 1968; Satterfield, 1973) as well as the historical development of the MBD concept, schools tend to call these children neurologically handicapped and, very often, make a neurological evaluation a prerequisite for the child's enrollment in a learning disability program. Moreover, it is not at all unusual for teachers to request directly that the neurologist place the child on an amphetamine or related compound.

A major task for the pediatric neurologist working with MBD children is to separate the essential from the nonessential, the primary from the secondary, and to outline a problem-oriented approach rather than one that merely yields a diagnostic label. In addition, he/she must work closely and productively in an advocacy role with parents, teachers, pediatricians, school psychologists, and, at times, other professionals as well.

Mental Retardation

Exact statistics about the total frequency and / or prevalence of mental retardation do not exist. However, an estimate of 3% in the school-age population is generally accepted. Of these, some 85% form the category of mild mental retardation with an IQ of 55 to 70. The etiology in this group appears to be multifactorial, and in the United States it is often assumed to be related to social cultural deprivation. Nevertheless, genetic and neurological factors are probably involved fairly frequently. For example, Benda (1964) calculated that about 20% of mentally retarded individuals with IQs higher than 55 can be expected to have some underlying pathology of the central nervous system. What is true in this population is that their mental handicap is usually less global than for moderately to profoundly retarded individuals. Therefore, assistance in early recognition (prior to school age) by the pediatric neurologist of specific weaknesses in higher functions of the CNS, such as impairment of memory functions, deficient speech and / or language, agnosias, apraxias, and impairment of abstract comprehension and thought processes, can accomplish prevention of a further compounding of such deficits as well as the initiation of compensatory habilitation management.

Surveys, reports, and studies regarding moderate, severe, and profound mental retardation are much more exact and detailed. Most of the studies agree that the incidence of severe mental handicap is about 3.6 per 1,000 among the child population beyond the age of 5 (Mackay, 1976). Most of the etiological categories associated with severe retardation would suggest that at one time or other these children will be seen by a pediatric neurologist for clarification of the medical diagnosis and involvement in management.

With regard to behavior disorders of retarded children, a finding of the Isle of Wight study is relevant (Rutter, Tizard, and Whitmore, 1970). In this study it was shown that children with various chronic neurological disorders and / or epilepsy showed rates of psychiatric disorder three or four times higher than those in the general population. In addition, it was found that the behavior characteristics of children with brain dysfunction and psychiatric disorder resembled those of control children with psychiatric disorder but no known organic abnormality of the brain. From this and other work (Ernhart et al., 1963; Schulman, Kaspar, and Throne, 1965) it may be concluded that, except for some very primitive patterns of disturbed behavior in the profoundly retarded, there is no one type of disturbed behavior that is specific for the child with brain disorder. Rather, it is suggested here that behavior disturbances of retarded children usually result from a discrepancy between the child's perceptual, cognitive, and / or motor limitations and the inappropriate environmental expectations and demands. The consulting neurologist must acquire the expertise to identify and define the dynamics of this interaction and to jointly plan and even initiate adequate intervention and management strategies with other professionals.

Cerebral Palsy

According to the data of the Perinatal Project of the National Institute of Neurological and Communication Disorders and Stroke, the prevalence for nonacquired cerebral palsy is 2.6 per 1,000 among 7-year-old children, increasing to 5.2 per 1,000 if acquired cases are also considered (Nelson, 1977). Cerebral palsy can be considered a prototype of developmental disability in that more often than not the affected child will experience problems in areas other than the primary deficit (Cruickshank, 1976).

Among all published reports on the intelligence of children with cerebral palsy, the New Jersey study has been the most conservative. Among the 1,000 children evaluated, 22.7% were in the IQ range of 70–89, and 48.8% were unequivocally retarded, more than half of these in the IQ range below 50 (Hopkins, Bice, and Colton, 1954). Of 80 children with cerebral palsy evaluated at the Newcomen Clinic at Guy's Hospital in London, 31% had definite and significant visual deficits (Robinson, 1975). Cruickshank, Hallahan, and Bice (1976) and Patel and Bharucha (1972) have demonstrated frequent and significant problems in spatial perception in children with cerebral palsy who have normal intelligence and minor motor involvement. It is likely that these deficits contribute to the development of problems in academic achievement. In addition, articulatory speech difficulties in cerebral palsy, at times so severe as to mimic profound mental retardation, range from a high of 60% in athetoids to a low of approximately 30% in the hemiplegic and the diplegic (Ingram, 1964). Finally, a manifest seizure disorder in cerebral palsy occurs with a frequency of 35%–60%, depending on the clinical category of motor impairment (Crothers and Paine, 1959; Perlstein, Gibbs, and Gibbs, 1947).

In summary, cerebral palsy represents a long-term management condition that requires an ongoing cooperation between professionals with a variety of knowledge and skills, including the pediatric neurologist.

Seizure Disorders

The incidence of seizure disorders among children in the United States is essentially based on estimates. According to a survey by Kurland (1959), the prevalence of epilepsy of all forms can be assumed to be 4.4 per 1,000 in the age group 10–19. Long-term sequelae to neonatal seizures, the prognosis for later intellectual development, and the need for early habilitative intervention depend largely on the underlying seizure etiology. Volpe (1973) has shown that out of 347 infants with neonatal seizures, 83% survived and 36% of these had neurological and/or mental sequelae.

However, in Keen and Lee's (1973) study of 83 cases available for long-term follow-up, 80% had motor handicaps, further seizures, or an IQ below 85. These children are clearly in need of anticipatory management with regard to a developmental compounding of their primary problems.

The frequency of significant mental handicap following uncomplicated febrile convulsions has been reported as 2.0%–7.7% in different studies (Ekholm and Miemiva, 1950; Frantzen et al., 1970; Keith, 1964). However, in a study of 50 twin pairs (17 monozygotic, 32 dizygotic, and 1 undetermined), there was an indication of a much higher frequency of mild intellectual impairment subsequent to febrile convulsions (Schiottz-Christensen and Bruhn, 1973). With regard to seizures difficult to control, Roden, Shapiro, and Lennox (1977) have reported from the Lafayette Clinic that no more than 23% of their patients carried a diagnosis "epilepsy only." Forty-eight percent had intellectual impairments, 54% displayed behavioral disturbances, and 10% had positive neurological findings.

Further evidence of problems associated with seizure disorders comes from the work of Holdsworth and Whitmore (1974) who found that among children with epilepsy attending regular schools in London, England, 31.2% were completing work on a level above average, 53.1% were keeping up with the control children at or below average, and 15.6% were falling seriously behind. Twenty-one percent presented behavior problems and in these the frequency of seizures appeared to be an important factor. Finally, Rutter, Graham, and Yule (1970) reported a frequency of 18% of 2 or more years of reading retardation in epileptic children of normal or above normal intelligence.

The possible effects of anti-epileptic drugs in nontoxic dosages upon behavior and learning are still poorly understood. Mild states of sedation, mood changes, excitement, irritability, aggressiveness, restlessness, hyperactivity, loss of drive, depression, euphoria, impairment of concentration, inhibition of cognitive functions, learning disability, and depression of memory functions, as well as beneficial psychotropic effects, have all been reported (Reynolds, 1973). At the same time there has been limited success of efforts to relate such effects more accurately to dosages and blood levels and to separate the drug effects from those of the underlying specific seizures and their frequency (Dalby, 1971; Grant, 1974; Guey et al., 1967; Mirsky and Kornetsky, 1964; Ounsted, 1955; Reynolds and Travers, 1974).

All of these facts would appear to assign to the pediatric neurologist a central role in what needs to be an essentially interdisciplinary treatment and management process of seizure disorders in children. It is, in fact, this approach that has been presented by Schain and Lamm (1977) in their model of comprehensive seizure management of children.

Meningitis and Encephalitis

The annual number of survivors from endemic neonatal and hemophilus meningitis in the United States has been estimated to be 12,900, with 412 suffering from epilepsy, 750 with deficits serious enough to consider institutionalization, and 3,340 incurring some type of neurological and/or mental handicap. That means that every fourth child leaving the hospital after a bout of meningitis is in need of some degree of habilitative management. Expressed in another way, presently 1 out of 200 infants becomes afflicted with this type of meningitis, and 1 in 430 will lose his/her neurological integrity after this encounter (Gotschlich, 1978). Additional research has clearly demonstrated that recovery from these and other infections of the CNS is likely to leave the child with any of a wide range of neurological and mental handicaps (Earnest et al., 1971; Fitzhardinge et al., 1974; Gamstorp and Klockhoff, 1974; Greenbaum and Lurie, 1948; Levy, 1959). Some of these sequelae manifest themselves later in more subtle psychosocial domains (see Sabatino and Cramblett, 1968).

Accordingly, and particularly in children who encounter a potentially devastating acute neurological disease, the pediatric neurologist — acting as primary care physician or as consultant — must pay as close attention to mild, subtle, or specific neurological deficits as to the gross and global impairments. In the milder manifestations, the child will be rendered vulnerable with regard to subsequent optimal development. In more severe instances associated with motor handicap and/or seizures, islands of relatively better preserved neurological functions may offer an opportunity for compensation. In both, the neurologist should be a prime mover and advocate for the child, particularly in cooperation with the parents.

Head Injury

The 1966–1967 survey of United States' households by the National Center for Health Statistics ascertained an annual prevalence of 614,000 head injuries (as defined by the World Health Organization International Classification of Diseases) sustained in the home, and of 180,000 head injuries by motor vehicles or other accidents outside the home in children under the age of 6. This amounts to a conservative estimate of an annual incidence of significant head injuries in 3.3% of the population of infants and young children (Caveness, 1970).

In closed head injury in children, it is generally assumed that recovery is rapid and complete (Deneker and Loefwing, 1958; Mealy, 1968). However, Naughton (1971) has called attention to the fact that even a minor reduction in cognitive functioning and changes in personality following closed head injury in children of previously superior intelligence may cause considerable emotional distress for the children, their parents, and their teachers (see also Dillon and Leopold, 1961; Fuld and Fisher, 1977).

Brink et al. (1970) have shown that attention to just the motor aspects of possible sequelae may be misleading with regard to the total disability picture of children who have experienced traumatic coma (see also Heiskanen and Kaste, 1974). In their 1- to 7-year follow-up study of 46 children who had experienced coma of an average duration of 7 weeks (median 4 weeks), only 29% retained clinically significant severe spastic or ataxic impairments and 13% had aphasic problems. However, even with only gross testing of intelligence (WISC or Stanford-Binet), 70% had an IQ below 85, and 35% had an IQ below 70. The rates rose to 86% and 60%, respectively, in those children that were less than 8 years old at the time of the trauma. Altogether, only 20% of all children were able to attend a regular school. In addition, personality and behavior problems were extremely common. The authors emphasize that recovery may occur for as long as 2 to 5 years, with a maximum in the first year. In support of proponents of early intervention, this period is when extensive rehabilitation efforts are both most promising and effective. Brink et al. (1970) recommend strongly that the physician attending the child during the acute phase of trauma and coma carry the obligation to initiate a rehabilitation process, including counseling of the parents, from the very beginning.

The Role of the Pediatric Neurologist: Summary

The following points are offered as a summary of this section with a number of important implications here drawn with regard to the role of the pediatric neurologist in the management of children with developmental disabilities.

1.   A majority of children with developmental problems suffer from non-progressive afflictions of the central nervous system. These range from the very mild, subtle, and/or specific to the severe, gross, and/or global.

2.   Owing to the unique properties of children as maturing, developing, and learning organisms, seemingly irreversible and stable neurological deficits have the potential to become compounded by malfunction in areas other than the primary deficit, as well as to respond favorably to efforts of modification, amelioration, and compensation. Which of the two will occur depends upon the nature and the quality of the long-term management. An appropriate management plan must include the child's home and school environment.

3.   Pediatric neurologists, as a rule, have been well-trained and have acquired the expertise to identify underlying impairments of the CNS.

They are able to recognize associated neurological functional deficits and to treat them *as long as they are in an acute stage.*

4.   However, a very sizable portion of the caseload of pediatric neurologists engaged in direct patient care consists of children with manifest or potential chronic developmental disabilities. If anything, this caseload can be expected to increase.

5.   More often than not, the evaluation and the long-term management of children with chronic developmental disabilities calls for the expertise and the active participation and cooperation of a variety of different child care professionals as part of an ongoing interdisciplinary process.

6.   Both the existing and predicted shortages in clinical pediatric neurological manpower, the complex nature of developmental disabilities, and the required long-term rehabilitation and habilitation process appear to render the pediatric neurologist most efficient in the role of a consultant.

7.   In order to be most effective as an interdisciplinary consultant, a great deal of flexibility is required. His/her role may range widely and may include leadership, guidance, coordination, or simply the provision of supportive participation in a team effort.

IMPLICATIONS FOR TRAINING

It is possible to identify at this time certain specific knowledge and clinical and technical skills as well as attitudes that should be maintained while evaluating children with developmental disabilities and planning for their long-term management. However, for purposes of this chapter, the following list is presented to provide an overview of these skills and abilities. It is certainly not intended that this list be comprehensive nor exhaustive, but it may be useful in highlighting key concepts that have emerged in relation to exceptional children and it may also be of value in guiding the development of training programs. Accordingly, it is suggested that the well-prepared pediatric neurologist in this area will be able to:

1.   Recognize and define the primary underlying impairment as accurately as possible.
2.   Separate the primary and irreversible from the secondary, preventable, and/or remediable.
3.   Recognize and define not only the weaknesses but also the strengths of the child, in particular those preserved areas of neurological integrity that can be amplified and utilized for the habilitation process.
4.   Be aware of and take into consideration the following: A certain and

still poorly understood amount of variability and unpredictability with regard to normal and deviant development exists. The complex processes of interaction between anatomic and functional CNS maturation in the presence of an organic deficit and the potential effects of future experience are still incompletely understood (Goldman, 1975; Isaacson, 1976; Provence, 1973; Touwen, 1978).

5. Be aware of and take into consideration the sum total of the child's environmental conditions, his/her ecosystem as it were.
6. Formulate a prognosis strictly within the confines of what can be prognosticated unequivocally.
7. Implement a problem-oriented approach with regard to long-term management.
8. Remain aware of one's own cognitive, attitudinal, and therapeutic limitations as well as the knowledge and the management potentials and skills of other child care disciplines.
9. Communicate with parents and other child care professionals on a basis of one's true knowledge and skills.
10. Remain considerate of the plight of the child's parents.

Residency Training

It is probably true that pediatric neurologists involved primarily in direct patient care can acquire some of the knowledge, skills, and attitudes essential for the interdisciplinary long-term management of children with developmental disabilities as they accumulate practical experience. However, appropriate supplementary training during the residency is to be preferred.

Presently, the American Board of Psychiatry and Neurology requires 2 years of general pediatric training and 3 years of neurology in an officially approved residency program to obtain certification in neurology with special competence in child neurology. Of the 2 years in pediatrics, one is specified as a PL-2 year (or its equivalent), as defined by the American Board of Pediatrics. Of the required 3 years in neurology, 1 year is defined as a neurological residency devoted to clinical child neurology and 1 year is devoted to adult clinical neurology. One year in pediatrics and 1 year in neurology are flexible. However, during the latter, emphasis is to be placed upon basic neurological sciences, closely related (medical) specialties, and special studies and laboratory procedures (*Directory of Accredited Residencies,* 1977).

At this writing the American Board of Psychiatry and Neurology requires only limited training in the developmental disabilities area for candidates seeking certification. However, in the Special Requirements for Residency Training in Child Neurology, mention is made of psychology, the neurology of learning, experience in problems dealing with growth and development of the normal child and adolescent, and the care of sick children, including those with mental retardation. Also, guidelines are provided through Part I of the written examination in the area of basic psychiatry, which addresses itself to normal and abnormal growth and development through the life cycle, including mental retardation. The written examination in the area of neurology covers mainly basic neurological sciences and diagnostic procedures.

Regarding the required PL-2 year in pediatrics, it would appear that future pediatric neurologists are given an adequate opportunity to familiarize themselves at least with the factual knowledge, the clinical, technical, and interpersonal skills, as well as the attitudes that are germane to the long-term management of chronic disabling conditions in childhood. However, the Task Force on Pediatric Education (1978) states unequivocally that, even within the 3-year pediatric curriculum:

> The educational content of many residency programs is inadequate...in ...the biosocial and developmental aspects of pediatrics (early adjustment problems and school failure as well as all those deriving from abnormal growth and development in the child who is chronically ill or is socially, mentally, or emotionally disturbed)...chronic illness...community pediatrics, handicapping and chronic conditions...and medical ethics (pp. 1 and 19).

It is extremely unlikely that, across the board, residents in pediatric neurology obtain this type of training exposure during their mandatory year in pediatric neurology. The time is just too short, and there is plainly too much physiological and clinical neurology to be learned that is different from adult neurology. In fact, Earnest (1978), speaking of the training in neurology in general, states that most programs

> ...emphasize inpatient care...services...in which patients are either acutely ill or have been referred for diagnostic evaluation of complex problems...the faculty [having] limited expertise in practicing and teaching general ambulatory care (p. 1).

Modifying the Curriculum

What then is the answer relative to the obvious training needs in the area of the long-term management of chronic neurological handicapping or developmental disabilities in children? Should there be an explicit portion of the curriculum devoted to mental retardation and other developmental disabilities? And if so, should it be placed into the pediatric or the neurological part of the residency? There are at this time no hard and fast answers.

As a specialty, pediatric neurology is still in its developmental stages. The definition of training content and objectives, as well as the formulation of the anticipated practice demands, continue to be subject to change

(Erenberg, 1978). This fact would appear to offer an excellent opportunity for an appropriate broadening of the scope of the residency training.

Certainly, pediatric neurologists are presently well trained with regard to the examination, evaluation, and diagnosis of neurological diseases in children and their management in the acute stages. However, as noted, the clinical judgment, skills, and attitudes necessary for the evaluation and long-term management of children with developmental disabilities with a view toward rehabilitation and habilitation are quite different. What is required is an opportunity for residents to witness and directly experience all of the interactions and processes essential for effective long-term management. It appears that programs of extended ambulatory care involving several disciplines (Medical Education and Medical Care: A Dynamic Equilibrium, 1973) are necessary to accomplish effective management.

The ambulatory setting provides an excellent opportunity for residents to learn their roles as members of the health care team. Involvement in this setting requires participation with other professionals including those from psychiatry and other medical specialties, social work, nursing, psychology, audiology, speech, occupational therapy, physical therapy, nutrition, and education — all of them being relevant to the habilitation of children with developmental disabilities. However, for such ambulatory settings to produce the desired results in terms of efficient training for the long-term management of handicapped children, certain modifications from the presently limited clinic models will have to take place. Such changes are likely to include clinic assignments for extended periods of time, regular chart reviews, case management conferences, encouragement and facilitation of applied research, and assignment to the clinical setting of full-time staff members who devote a majority of time to ambulatory care and teaching. In addition, practical, constructive, and productive interactions and cooperation with other child care professionals from both the clinical setting and the community are essential (Earnest, 1978).

Similar training issues are presently being considered by the American Academy of Pediatrics and the American Board of Pediatrics. Whether residents in pediatric neurology will be exposed to an in-depth experience in developmental disabilities during their training in pediatrics may actually depend on the point in time at which such a training opportunity will be placed into the standard pediatric curriculum; that is to say, prior to PL-3. The fact that the American Board of Psychiatry and Neurology has left 1 of the 2 years required in pediatrics completely flexible would appear to offer to residents in pediatric neurology a realistic opportunity to avail themselves of the anticipated training experiences in developmental disabilities during that time.

Such training could certainly not be accommodated during the required year in adult neurology, and it could only be accommodated with difficulty during that year in pediatric neurology. However, although the Board has established a number of requirements relative to the contents of the third year in neurology, there is nevertheless some degree of flexibility.

An appropriate exposure relative to the future work of the pediatric neurologist with developmentally disabled children could be arranged within settings such as seizure, neuromuscular, learning disability, cerebral palsy, physical medicine, blind and deaf, or high risk infant clinics. In addition, there are now various clinical evaluation, rehabilitation, habilitation and/or school programs attached to some 40 University Affiliated Facilities throughout the country focusing on mental retardation and other developmental disabilities. These training programs are designed and equipped to demonstrate and to teach the factual knowledge, technical skills, clinical judgment, interpersonal skills, and attitudes that should enable the pediatric neurologist to be optimally effective and efficient in caring for developmentally disabled children within an interdisciplinary model. As a rule, residents rotating through any of these facilities experience the gratification of being able to teach other disciplines as much as they learn from them.

A number of the necessary clinical practice requirements associated with the preventive and long-term management of developmentally disabled children and their families were touched upon in earlier sections of this chapter. Additional details can be found in a variety of other sources (e.g., Apley, 1978; Koch and Kugel, 1971). Furthermore, as illustrated in the various chapters of this volume, development of specific curriculum components in the area of developmental disabilities for pediatric residents and the evaluation of their effectiveness is just beginning, but the charge is unequivocal and the urgency is great.

REFERENCES

Apley, J. (Ed.). 1978. Care of the Handicapped Child. Clinics in Developmental Medicine, No. 67. London: William Heinman Medical Books.
Benda, C. C. 1964. Die geistigen entwicklungsstoerungen in kindersalter. Der Nervearzt, 35, 97–101.
Bergström, K., and Bille, B. 1978. Computed tomography of the brain in children with minimal brain damage: A preliminary study of 46 children. Neuropädiatric, 9, 378–384.
Bresnan, M. H., Nakano, K. K., and Snodgrass, S. R. 1976. Medical Examination Review Vol. 35, Pediatric Neurology. Flushing, N.Y.: Medical Examination Publishing Company, Inc.

Brink, J. D., Garret, A. L., Hale, W. R., Woo-Sam, J., and Nickel, V. L. 1970. Recovery of motor and intellectual function in children sustaining severe head injuries. Developmental Medicine and Child Neurology, 12, 565–571.

Capute, A. J., Niedermeyer, E. F. L., and Richardson, F. 1968. The electro-encephalogram in children with minimal cerebral dysfunction. Pediatrics, 41, 1104–1115.

Carter, S. 1971. Of priorities, promise and the path ahead. Neurology, 21, 877–888.

Caveness, W. 1970. Epidemiologic studies of head injury. In C. R. Augle and E. A. Bering (Eds.), Physical Trauma as an Etiological Agent in Mental Retardation. Proceedings of a Conference on the Etiology of Mental Retardation.

Crothers, B., and Paine, R. S. 1959. The Natural History of Cerebral Palsy. London: Oxford University Press.

Cruickshank, W. M. 1976. The problem and its scope. In W. M. Cruickshank (Ed.), Cerebral Palsy. Syracuse: Syracuse University Press.

Cruickshank, W. M., and Hallahan, D. P., with Bice, H. V. 1976. The evaluation of intelligence. In W. M. Cruickshank (Ed.), Cerebral Palsy. Syracuse: Syracuse University Press.

Dalby, M. A. 1971. Antiepileptic and psychotropic effects of carbamazepine (Tegretol) in the treatment of psychomotor epilepsy. Epilepsia, 12, 325–334.

Deneker, S. J., and Loefwing, B. 1958. A psychometric study of identical twins discordant for closed head injury. ACTA Psychiatrica and Neurologica Scandinavica, 33, suppl. 122.

Dillon, H., and Leopold, R. L. 1961. Children and the postconcussion syndrome. Journal of the American Medical Association, 175, 86–92.

Directory of Accredited Residencies. 1977. Chicago: American Medical Association.

Earnest, M. P. 1978. Ambulatory neurology in residency training programs: A perspective. Neurology, 28, 1–4.

Earnest, M. P., Goolishian, H. A., Calverley, J. R., Hayes, R. O., and Hill, M. R. 1971. Neurologic, intellectual, and psychologic sequelae following western encephalitis. Neurology, 21, 969–974.

Eisenberg, L. 1966. Reading retardation. I. Psychiatric and sociological aspects. Pediatrics, 37, 352–365.

Ekholm, E., and Miemiva, K. 1950. On convulsions in early childhood and their prognosis. ACTA Paediatrica (Uppsala), 39, 481–501.

Erenberg, G. 1978. Personal communication.

Ernhart, C. B., Graham, F. K., Eichman, P. L., Marshall, J. M., and Thurston, D. 1963. Brain injury in the pre-school child: Some developmental considerations. II. Comparison of brain-injured and normal children. Psychological Monographs, 77 (No. 11).

Fitzhardinge, P. M., Kazemi, M., Ramsay, M., and Stern, L. 1974. Long-term sequelae of neonatal meningitis. Developmental Medicine and Child Neurology, 16, 3–10.

Frantzen, E., Lennox-Buchthal, M. A., Nygaard, A., and Stene, J. 1970. A genetic study of febrile convulsions. Neurology, 20, 909–917.

Fuld, P. A., and Fisher, P. 1977. Recovery of intellectual ability after closed head injury. Developmental Medicine and Child Neurology, 19, 495–502.

Gamstorp, I., and Klockhoff, I. 1974. Bilateral, severe sensori-neural hearing loss after haemophilus influenzae meningitis in childhood. Neuropaediatrie, 5, 121–124.

Goldman, P. S. 1975. Age, sex, and experience as related to the neurologic basis of cognitive development. In N. A. Buchwald and M. A. B. Brazier (Eds.), Brain Mechanisms in Mental Retardation. New York: Academic Press, Inc.

Gotschlich, E. C. 1978. Vaccines for Bacterial Meningitis (Plan for Nationwide Action on Epilepsy, Vol. II, Part 2, p. 295). Washington, D.C.: U.S. Department of Health, Education and Welfare.

Grant, R. H. E. 1974. Sulthamine and behavior. Developmental Medicine and Child Neurology, 16, 821-824.

Greenbaum, J. V., and Lurie, L. A. 1948. Encephalitis as a causative factor in behavior disorders of children. Journal of the American Medical Association, 136, 923-930.

Guey, J., Charles, C., Coquery, C., Roger, S., and Soulayrol, R. 1967. Study of psychological effects of ethosuximide (Zarontin) on 25 children suffering from petit mal epilepsy. Epilepsia, 8, 129-141.

Hagbert, B., Ingram, T. T. S., and MacKeith, R. 1970. Development of pediatric neurology. The Lancet, 1, 940-942.

Heiskanen, O., and Kaste, M. 1974. Late prognosis of severe brain injury in children. Developmental Medicine and Child Neurology, 16, 11-14.

Holdsworth, L., and Whitmore, K. 1974. A study of children with epilepsy attending ordinary schools. Developmental Medicine and Child Neurology, 16, 746-758.

Hopkins, T., Bice, H. V., and Colton, K. C. 1954. Evaluation and Education of the Cerebral Palsied Child — New Jersey Study. Washington, D.C.: International Council for Exceptional Children.

Ingram, T. T. S. 1964. Pediatric Aspects of Cerebral Palsy. London: E. and S. Livingstone Ltd.

Isaacson, R. L. 1976. Recovery (?) from early brain damage. In T. D. Tjossem (Ed.), Intervention Strategies for High Risk Infants and Young Children. Baltimore: University Park Press.

Keen, J. H., and Lee, D. 1973. Sequelae of neonatal convulsions. Archives of Diseases of Childhood, 48, 542-546.

Keith, H. M. 1964. Convulsions in children under 3 years of age: A study of prognosis. Proceedings of the Staff Meetings of the Mayo Clinic, 39, 895-907.

Koch, R., and Kugel, R. B., (Eds.). 1971. The pediatrician and the child with mental retardation. Evanston, Ill.: American Academy of Pediatrics.

Kurland, L. T. 1959. The incidence and prevalence of convulsive disorders in a small urban community. Epilepsia (Amsterdam), 4, 142-161.

Levy, S. 1959. Postencephalitic behavior disorders: A forgotten entity. American Journal of Psychiatry, 115, 1062-1067.

Mackay, R. J. 1976. Mental Handicap in Child Health Practice. London: Butterworths.

Mealy, J. 1968. Pediatric Head Injuries. Springfield, Ill.: Charles C Thomas Publisher.

Medical education and medical care: A dynamic equilibrium. 1973. Proceedings of a Fogarty International Center Conference. Journal of Medical Education, 48, 51-73.

Mirsky, A. F., and Kornetsky, C. 1964. On the dissimilar effects of drugs on the digit symbol substitution and continuous performance tests. Psychopharmacologia, 5, 161-177.

Naughton, J. A. L. 1971. The effects of severe head injuries in children: Psychological aspects. In Proceedings of an International Symposium on Head Injuries, April 2-10, 1970. Edinburgh: Churchill-Livingston.

Nelson, K. 1977. The epidemiology of cerebral palsy. Paper presented at the Conference on the Epidemiology of Neurological Disorders of the National Institute of Neurological and Communication Disorders and Stroke and Georgetown University Medical School, Washington, D.C.

Ounsted, C. 1955. The hyperkinetic syndrome in epileptic children. The Lancet, 303-311.

Patel, S., and Bharucha, E. P. 1972. The Bender-Gestalt test as a measure of perceptual and visuo-motor defects in cerebral palsied children. Developmental Medicine and Child Neurology, 14, 156-160.

Pearson, G. H. J. 1952. A survey of learning difficulties in children. Psychoanalytic Study of the Child, 7, 322-386.

Perlstein, M. A., Gibbs, E. L., and Gibbs, F. A. 1947. The electroencephalogram in infantile cerebral palsy. Proceedings in Research of Nervous and Mental Diseases, 26, 377-384.

Provence, S. 1973. Therapeutic intervention: What constitutes intervention in the early years? In F. Richardson (Ed.), Brain and Intelligence. Hyattsville, Md.: National Educational Press.

Reynolds, E. H. 1973. Chronic anticonvulsants and toxicity — A review. Proceedings of XII International Congress on Epilepsy. Barcelona, Spain.

Reynolds, E. H., and Travers, R. D. 1974. Serum anticonvulsant concentrations in epileptic patients with mental symptoms. British Journal of Psychiatry, 124, 440-445.

Robinson, R. O. 1975. The frequency of other handicaps in children with cerebral palsy. Developmental Medicine and Child Neurology, 15, 305-312.

Roden, E. A., Shapiro, H. L., and Lennox, K. 1977. Epilepsy and life performance. Rehabilitation Literature, 38, 34-39.

Rutter, M., Graham, P., and Yule, B. 1970. A Neuropsychiatric Study in Childhood. London: Spastics International Medical Publications with William Heineman Medical Books.

Rutter, M., Tizard, J., and Whitmore, K. 1970. Education, Health and Behavior. New York: John Wiley & Sons, Inc.

Sabatino, D. A., and Cramblett, H. G. 1968. Behavioral sequelae of California encephalitis virus infection in children. Developmental Medicine and Child Neurology, 10, 331-337.

Satterfield, J. H. 1973. EEG issues in children with minimal brain dysfunction. In S. Walzer and P. H. Wolff (Eds.), Minimal Brain Dysfunction in Children. New York: Grune & Stratton.

Schain, R. J., and Lamm, C. 1977. Comprehensive management of children with seizure disorders. Paper presented at the 31st annual meeting of the American Academy for Cerebral Palsy and Developmental Medicine, October 5-9, 1977, Atlanta.

Schiottz-Christensen, E., and Bruhn, P. 1973. Intelligence, behavior and scholastic achievement subsequent to febrile convulsions: An analysis of discordant twin pairs. Developmental Medicine and Child Neurology, 15, 565-575.

Schulman, J. L., Kaspar, J. C., and Throne, F. M. 1965. Brain Damage and Behaviour. A Clinical Experimental Study. Springfield, Ill.: Charles C Thomas Publisher.

Swaiman, K. F. 1974. Presidential address at the child neurology society. Developmental Medicine and Child Neurology, 16, 808-811.

The Task Force on Pediatric Education. 1978. The future of pediatric education. Evanston, Ill.: American Academy of Pediatrics.

Tibbles, J. A. R. 1976. The functions and the training of a pediatric neurologist. Developmental Medicine and Child Neurology, 18, 167–172.

Touwen, B. 1978. Variability and stereotype in normal and deviant development. In J. Apley (Ed.), Care of the Handicapped Child. Clinics in Developmental Medicine, No. 67. London: William Heineman Medical Books.

Volpe, J. 1973. Neonatal seizures. New England Journal of Medicine, 289, 413–416.

Weichsel, M. E., Jr. 1974. Child neurology in the community hospital setting. Pediatrics, 53, 895–899.

Wender, P. 1971. Minimal Brain Dysfunction in Children. New York: Wiley-Interscience.

Yahr, M. D. 1975. Summary report of the joint commission on neurology. Neurology, 25, 497–501.

FRAMEWORK FOR FUTURE EFFORTS

chapter 16

A COMPREHENSIVE CURRICULUM IN CHILD DEVELOPMENT AND HANDICAPPING CONDITIONS
Prospects for Design, Implementation, and Evaluation

H. Burtt Richardson, Jr., Michael J. Guralnick, Lawrence T. Taft, and Melvin D. Levine

An underlying theme of this book and the Conference on Pediatric Education and the Needs of Young Exceptional Children upon which it was based is that it is essential to define and introduce a comprehensive curriculum on the developmental needs of children with and without handicaps into pediatric curricula. Furthermore, it appears that in order to design, implement, and evaluate a curriculum, the pooling of the diverse backgrounds and competencies of pediatricians, psychologists, educators, and professionals from numerous other disciplines is essential. Such interdisciplinary collaboration, so crucial for the provision of adequate services to developing children, is equally crucial for the development and evaluation of pediatric educational efforts.

   The principles underlying pediatric education in the areas of child development and handicapping conditions are reviewed in the chapters of the first section of this book, and the experience with implementation and evaluation at various levels is presented in the second section. The purpose of this chapter is to summarize the goals and content areas of a possible comprehensive curriculum in child development and handicapping conditions, to discuss some practical constraints on curriculum design and implementation, and to describe an approach to curriculum evaluation. The outline of this proposed curriculum, its content, its implementation techniques, and especially its evaluation strategies draw upon the material presented in the previous chapters. Many themes, such as the essential role of the interdisciplinary process and the transactional approach to understanding the development of exceptional children, have emerged time and again. Similarly, the application of the tasks-by-abilities matrix in evaluating competencies has been described and implemented in various ways. In addition to these ideas and concepts, our view of a curriculum and its implementation was influenced by the vigorous discussion that accompanied the conference presentations. Some of the key ideas of the discussants are presented in the next section of this chapter, which is followed by sections on the content of a comprehensive curriculum, its design and implementation, and finally, its evaluation.

SUMMARY OF DISCUSSANTS' COMMENTS

The following summary of discussants' comments was prepared from transcripts of conference proceedings (see Preface).

There is some urgency in bringing pediatricians into an active and useful role in providing guidance in child development and oversight for the special needs of handicapped children. Parents no longer accept the, "He'll grow out of it," advice and indeed are often bitter about the apparent disinterest or lack of helpfulness of their child's doctor. Pediatrics must change through residents acquiring the skills and attitudes necessary to meet children's and parents' needs so that the public can regain justifiable confidence in the pediatrician's contribution. Such a contribution, of course, must be a collaborative one with other child development and educational professionals. The pediatrician must learn to contribute to, not insist on controlling or even necessarily leading, team efforts.

Resident education in this area, as in all others, requires "hands on" clinical experience and continuity of follow-up in order to have a permanent impact on the pediatrician's subsequent attitudes and clinical performance. Clinical experience with families as they cope with handicapped children is as important in the long run as is experience with the children themselves. If one accepts the premise that a pediatrician's future practices are influenced by residency experiences in clinical settings, it is vital to expose residents to programs aimed at early diagnosis, case-finding, referral for further study, and intervention.

There are certain practical issues that were emphasized by discussants in relation to the design and implementation of a residency curriculum in child development and handicapping conditions. First, the teaching of how a pediatrician should serve a handicapped child in practice is not complete if the resident is exposed only to the multidisciplinary University Affiliated Facility approach. Time needs to be devoted to the logistics of service in different settings, including those similar to office pediatric practice. Quality service/training programs are expensive, however, no matter what the setting. Funds, principally federal, must be sought if the resident's experience is to be of high quality.

To develop quality service in educational settings, pediatric department chairpersons and pediatric training program directors must see child development and handicapping conditions as a high priority within their overall budgets. The major responsibility, however, falls on the pediatrician who specializes in these fields. Neurologists and psychiatrists, who also deal frequently with developmentally handicapped children, should increasingly gain experience during their training from pediatric specialists. Too often, pediatric training program directors have delegated responsibility for teaching in this area to nonpediatric faculty members whose training and experience are inappropriate to deal with the comprehensive needs of the handicapped child.

The pediatric faculty member responsible for implementing a curriculum in child development and handicapping conditions must establish credibility with other department members. In academic settings, research is crucial for such acceptance. An area of research appropriate for such faculty members is the evaluation of the learning of medical students and pediatric residents. In spite of its importance to all pediatric faculty members, and indeed to pediatrics and medicine as a whole, relatively little is known about such learning processes. The evaluation of the effectiveness of clinical intervention is another area in which the developmental pediatrician can contribute with original research.

CONTENT OF A COMPREHENSIVE CURRICULUM

A comprehensive curriculum in child development and handicapping conditions might consist of the following 12 goals. These goals were designed within the framework of residency level training, but have implications for other levels as well. Each goal is presented as a competency statement. Also described are examples of specific content for each to be used to form subgoals and specific educational objectives.

1. *The participants will learn the basic principles, processes, and developmental milestones within the area of CHILD DEVELOPMENT.*

This goal focuses on the processes and stages of normal development and includes physical, motor, language, social, and emotional aspects. It is expected that residents will learn the principles and methods of child-rearing, will gain a recognition of the importance of sociocultural influences on child development, and will become able to view the child as a member of an ecological system consisting of immediate family, extended family, and community. Phenomena such as mother-infant bonding and other aspects of attachment as well as the relationship of the physical environment (for instance, toys or noise) and the transactional model of child development are also included.

2. *The participants will develop more positive ATTITUDES TO-WARD EXCEPTIONAL CHILDREN.* The curriculum content that leads pediatric residents to accepting exceptional children as patients revolves around direct clinical experience. It is also suggested that providing residents with an historical perspective of services for exceptional children leads to a clearer understanding and acceptance of current efforts in this regard. The resident is expected, however, to develop a working relationship with individual handicapped children including the opportunity to follow them as they develop in appropriate settings. Residents should also learn the implications of labels and the bill of rights for the mentally retarded.

3. *The participants will improve the level of their factual knowledge of HANDICAPPING CONDITIONS.* Included within this goal is the basic fund of knowledge that a pediatrician is expected to have regarding all handicaps, including sensory, physical, mental, and emotional ones. The resident should be familiar with the incidence, etiology, clinical manifestations, and natural course of major and minor conditions associated with handicaps. This includes all conditions associated with mental retardation, cerebral palsy, emotional disturbance, and specific learning disabilities. The resident is also expected to be able to classify handicaps by type and degree.

4. *The participants will learn the current methods of PREVENTION with regard to handicapping conditions.* Because of its particular importance and relevance to pediatrics, the prevention of handicapping conditions has been separated from the preceding goal. It is expected that residents should be aware of preventive aspects of genetic and chromosomal conditions, such as phenylketonuria and Down's syndrome; congenital conditions, such as fetal alcohol syndrome, fetal infections, and hypothyroidism; perinatal conditions, such as anoxia and intraventricular hemorrhage; and postnatal conditions, such as cerebral trauma, child abuse, and central nervous system infections. In addition to prevention on an individual basis,

residents should be familiar with approaches to the prevention of handicapping conditions for large populations. Current data, for instance, indicate that the implementation of neonatal intensive care on a regional basis reduces not only infant mortality but also the frequency of handicapping conditions in survivors. Similarly, regional approaches to amniocentesis, fetal monitoring, and metabolic screening will be implemented to the extent that residents are aware of their effectiveness in preventing handicaps. Distribution of the broad range of physical and mental health services to appropriate populations can also influence the frequency of handicaps, such as those resulting from accidents, meningitis, child abuse, and fetal alcohol syndrome.

5. *The participants will learn the use of SCREENING, DIAGNOSTIC, and ASSESSMENT procedures.* In order to participate in the identification and management of children with handicaps, pediatricians must gain knowledge of various screening and diagnostic instruments within pediatric psychology and education. They must, of course, be able to carry out the appropriate history, physical, and neurological examinations expected of them as members of a management team and, furthermore, should be able to apply certain specific screening or diagnostic instruments in clinical settings. As part of this goal, the resident must gain a perspective of the requirements for and the shortcomings of an adequate screening program; he/she must be aware of the tentative nature of diagnosis and of the need for the ongoing assessment of handicaps; and he/she must recognize his/her importance to the individual child. Furthermore, the interaction between assessment and remediation must be seen by the pediatrician evaluating a child's learning. It is important that the most prevalent handicapping conditions, such as mild handicaps and learning disabilities, be given particular weight in this aspect of the pediatric resident's curriculum.

6. *The participants will learn to function effectively as members of an INTERDISCIPLINARY TEAM.* Residents must be exposed to members of a variety of disciplines and must learn the particular roles and contributions of the discipline. For the resident entering practice, the indications for seeking consultation and the ability to understand and utilize the skills and knowledge of members of different disciplines is crucial to the adequate management of a child with handicaps. It is also in the context of interdisciplinary team membership that the pediatric resident can perhaps best learn elements of group process particularly as it relates to leadership within a group. Furthermore, residents must develop adequate communication with classroom teachers, school counselors, administrators,

and other school system professionals. Communication of behavioral and social, as well as medical, information to colleagues in nonmedical disciplines must be learned; the resident must have opportunity for both oral and written communication of such information.

7. *The participant will learn his/her role in the MANAGEMENT of handicapping conditions.* As an individual or team member, the pediatrician is responsible for initiating diagnostic and treatment efforts for any conditions amenable to medical therapy and often has a further coordinating responsibility for many other nonmedical therapies, particularly in the preschool child. Learning management responsibilities will probably require a resident's participation in the longitudinal management of a variety of handicapped children. In this way residents can learn to cope with some of the problems inherent in managing chronic conditions that are resistant to marked change.

8. *The participants will learn to communicate effectively with PARENTS of handicapped children.* This aspect of the resident's curriculum includes how to obtain factual and interpersonal information from parents, how to counsel parents with regard to the instructional needs of the child, and how to provide genetic counseling. In addition, residents should be aware of the social and financial implications of a handicapped child on the family and should be able to carry out long-range planning with the parents concerning the child's developmental and educational needs. An awareness of the importance of parents' groups for learning and support should also be included in the curriculum.

9. *The participants will become more knowledgeable about COMMUNITY RESOURCES and more skillful in using them to meet the needs of individual handicapped children and their families.* Included in this goal is an understanding of criteria for referral to various local facilities, the relationship between private and public (state and local) agencies, and the differences between resources for children with single and multiple handicaps. The resident should gain experience in selecting community resources, responding to the needs of the agencies and the children, and coordinating the referral process when appropriate. Special emphasis should be placed on understanding the role of the public school system in the particular community. The resident should be familiar with the special educational interventions that are available and the administrative procedures for individual children with learning problems or more severe handicaps, particularly with regard to Public Law 94-142.

10. *The participants will become more knowledgeable and skillful in providing general HEALTH AND MEDICAL CARE for handi-*

capped children. This aspect of the curriculum presents the distinction between medical and educational models and the appropriate use of both for providing services to handicapped children. Health promotion as well as the diagnosis and remediation of medical conditions often found among the handicapped is emphasized. The resident should also be offered the opportunity to become familiar with school health services and school policies regarding physical handicaps and medications.

11. *The participants will become more aware of classical and recent DE-VELOPMENTAL, EDUCATIONAL, AND PSYCHOLOGICAL RESEARCH.* Residents should become as familiar with the scientific basis for educational/developmental interventions as they are for medical treatments. The studies, as they become available, documenting the effectiveness of early intervention, the rationale for various educational approaches, and the documentation of educational outcomes should be included. It is important that residents become familiar with accepted practices within education and psychology and gain some awareness of current controversies within these fields and related disciplines.

12. *The participants will become more aware of LEGAL AND LEGISLATIVE ASPECTS of handicapping conditions.* The resident must be prepared to understand the pediatrician's role in the implementation of the Education for All Handicapped Children Act (Public Law 94-142), and he/she should understand the related concepts of least restrictive environment and individual educational plans as well as the respective rights and duties of schools, teachers, and parents. The pediatrician's role as a children's advocate in promoting improved school policies and legislation in the interest of all children, including the handicapped, should also be included in the residents' curriculum.

CURRICULUM DESIGN AND IMPLEMENTATION

Each of the curriculum goal areas just described can be further divided into subgoals and specific objectives to be accomplished in the context of a particular learning activity. Such activities can be quite varied and will differ with the resources available. In order to ensure flexibility of the curriculum, particular objectives should be designed so that they may be met with the residents' experiencing any of a number of activities. Examples of activities available for different aspects of the curriculum include reading, audiovisual presentation, lectures or seminars, observation in various clinical or educational settings, simulated clinical activities, and direct clinical experience with children, school personnel, and interdisciplinary teams.

The time available for teaching child development and handicapping conditions is quite variable among different pediatric training programs. It is recommended that a core set of activities totalling 160 hours or a 1-month rotation at the residency level be a minimum requirement. These learning activities should be keyed to overall goals and objectives, such as those described in the preceding section of this chapter. The core curriculum can be supplemented by additional, in-depth activities for residents with particular interests in this aspect of pediatrics or for residency programs where more than 1 month is allocated to child development and handicapping conditions.

The choice of the particular activities for accomplishing the curriculum goals depends on: 1) the number of residents available to participate in a program at any one time, 2) the time available for faculty members to participate in direct resident teaching, and, perhaps most importantly, 3) the availability of children and their parents served by members of an interdisciplinary team. Regardless of the particular clinical resources available, the designers of the resident curriculum should provide for a variety of clinical experiences that parallel the variety of resources in different community settings (from the rural pediatric practitioner's office to the child development unit of a University Affiliated Facility). Ideally, the pediatric resident could then learn the skill of bringing together scarce resources for the benefit of an individual handicapped child, as well as the skill of maintaining a rational child-oriented approach while gathering appropriate resources from those potentially available in a major university center.

The definition of specific educational activities relating to curriculum objectives allows for application of portions of the curriculum to students at other levels than the residency level. For instance, certain introductory aspects of child development and handicapping conditions may be appropriate within a particular pediatric department for all medical students; indeed some with special interests may complete the core pediatric residency curriculum prior to graduation from medical school. Finally, the availability of supplementary activities in each curriculum goal area would provide the opportunity for development of further depth and breadth of knowledge and skills for the interested resident and can also provide direction for further training for pediatricians entering specialty fellowships following their core of pediatric resident years.

CURRICULUM EVALUATION

Subjective approaches to curriculum evaluation are well known to all pediatric training program directors as residents provide feedback regarding what they like or dislike and what they find valuable. Faculty members indicate by their participation, or lack of it, what they find of practical value in teaching residents. A valid evaluation of the effectiveness of a curriculum, however, depends on a more objective assessment of improved knowledge, skills, attitudes, or clinical judgment on the part of the residents participating in the curriculum. As stressed throughout virtually every chapter of this book, the process of specifying curriculum objectives in terms that are amenable to measurement is essential in order to evaluate a curriculum's effectiveness.

Evaluation measures during the training program can include: 1) multiple choice and other written or oral tests of knowledge, 2) written or oral checklists of skills or attitudes, 3) direct observation of interpersonal and technical skills, and 4) patient management problems for the assessment of clinical judgment. In fact, it may be possible to use computer technology to design patient management problems, which include multiple choice questions and attitude or skill assessment for the various educational objectives.

The organization and evaluation of a curriculum in child development and handicapping conditions can be similar to that of other aspects of pediatric practice. For instance, the model developed by the American Board of Pediatrics (*Foundations for Evaluating the Competency of Pediatricians,* 1974), which divides the clinical problem-solving process into abilities and tasks has been described in a number of chapters (see Chapter 6, this volume for details) as being relevant to a child development and handicapped child curriculum.

Since this approach has been stressed in this book, although there are other viable and interesting models for curriculum design and evaluation (e.g., see Chapter 5, this volume), the 12 curriculum goals suggested in this chapter were distributed in relation to the tasks-by-abilities matrix. This was accomplished by the authors examining each of the goals and the general content for each and determining whether a given cell applies. Although somewhat arbitrary, it did serve to highlight certain patterns. For convenience, the tasks-by-abilities matrix is reproduced in Figure 1. Please note that the term *development* was added to the third task.

Table 1 presents the distribution of the 12 curriculum goals among the 15 cells of the matrix. Inspection of the table reveals that a substantial number of goals require evaluation with regard to factual knowledge and attitudes. On the other hand, technical skills are associated with only two goals. Consequently, for residents who expect that technical skills development will be emphasized here as it is in other rotations, certain problems can result. Of course, all goals are not given equal weight in terms of time and resources, but possible differences and potential problems be-

Tasks

Abilities	1—Gathering, organizing and recording data	2—Assessing data	3—Managing problems and maintaining health and development
A—Attitudes	A1	A2	A3
B—Factual knowledge	B1	B2	B3
C—Interpersonal skills	C1	C2	C3
D—Technical skills	D1	D2	D3
E-Clinical judgment	E1	E2	E3

Figure 1.   Matrix associating tasks and abilities. Adapted from the American Board of Pediatrics, Inc. 1974. Reprinted by permission.

tween a core curriculum for a rotation in child development and handicapping conditions and other rotations should not be minimized.

Since effective problem-solving in clinical situations with handicapped children and their families from diagnosis through long-term management is an overriding goal of the training program, it is possible to utilize the tasks-by-abilities matrix as both a tool for summative evaluation and as a means of identifying content. At a practical level, summative evaluation of clinical problem-solving of this magnitude is difficult to carry out. The complexity and time required for the task is simply too extensive and, for a summative evaluation, it would be expected to occur following completion of the training program. One possible solution is to simulate this process through computer-assisted patient management problems. The problem can be programmed based on content derived from the matrix. Sufficiently sophisticated technology exists to permit interactive sequences to be programmed that are able to capture the temporal and integrative aspects of the clinical problem-solving process. Of course, there are a number of abilities and tasks that are not amenable to this form of evaluation, but it stands as an interesting and potentially valuable approach to the evaluation of a complex problem.

This use of the tasks-by-abilities matrix as applied to the handicapped child and his/her family can perhaps be seen more clearly by providing an example of a clinical problem. The details of a situation in which a pediatrician is presented with the case of a pregnant mother who already has a Down's syndrome child are presented in the Appendix to this chapter. Relevant tasks and abilities have been identified, although it is not intended that this example be exhaustive with respect to the competencies required in each cell for effective solution of the problem. In addition, the information is ordered in terms of goal number rather than chronological sequence as would occur in the actual problem-solving process. With further development, the information contained within each cell of the matrix can be related to a specific educational objective within each goal area of the curriculum. Consequently, successful completion of the core curriculum, in this example, would provide the pediatric resident with sufficient information, skills, attitudes, and clinical judgment to approach this problem in the most professional way possible.

Finally, it should be noted that the process of devising competency matrices for significant clinical problems can serve as a basis for identifying content that may have been omitted from the original curriculum. That is, if a tasks-by-abilities matrix is developed for a new but significant clinical situation, yet certain skills or abilities identified in the cells to solve this problem were not part of the goals and educational objectives, modification of the curriculum content and associated activities can be carried out.

Table 1. Relationship of curriculum goals to evaluation matrix

Abilities	Data gathering	Assessment	Management
Attitudes	1. Child development 2. Attitudes toward exceptional children 4. Prevention 6. Interdisciplinary team 12. Legal and legislative aspects	1. Child development 2. Attitudes toward exceptional children 4. Prevention 6. Interdisciplinary team 12. Legal and legislative aspects	1. Child development 2. Attitudes toward exceptional children 4. Prevention 6. Interdisciplinary team 7. Management 12. Legal and legislative aspects
Factual knowledge	1. Child development 3. Handicapping conditions 4. Prevention 5. Screening, diagnostic, assessment 6. Interdisciplinary team 9. Community resources	1. Child development 3. Handicapping conditions 4. Prevention 5. Screening, diagnostic, assessment 6. Interdisciplinary team 9. Community resources	1. Child development 3. Handicapping conditions 4. Prevention 6. Interdisciplinary team 7. Management 9. Community resources

	10. Health and medical care 11. Developmental, educational, and psychological research 12. Legal and legislative aspects 6. Interdisciplinary team 8. Parents 10. Health and medical care	10. Health and medical care 11. Developmental, educational, and psychological research 12. Legal and legislative aspects 6. Interdisciplinary team 8. Parents 10. Health and medical care	10. Health and medical care 11. Developmental, educational, and psychological research 12. Legal and legislative aspects 6. Interdisciplinary team 7. Management 8. Parents 10. Health and medical care 10. Health and medical care
Interpersonal skills			
Technical skills	5. Screening, diagnostic, assessment 10. Health and medical care	5. Screening, diagnostic, assessment 10. Health and medical care	
Clinical judgment	6. Interdisciplinary team 8. Parents 10. Health and medical care	6. Interdisciplinary team 8. Parents 10. Health and medical care	6. Interdisciplinary team 7. Management 8. Parents 9. Community resources 10. Health and medical care

197

CONCLUSIONS

The rationale, constraints, potential educational strategies and content for the design, implementation, and evaluation of a curriculum in child development and handicapping conditions are described. The press by virtually every concerned professional and consumer group for increased and systematic efforts in the area of pediatric education and the needs of exceptional children, as well as the consistent themes that have emerged, attest to the significance of this issue. Finally, we wish to point out that should such a coordinated national effort be forthcoming, it will mark another important historical event in professional training related to exceptional children and their families — an area that has previously been at the periphery of many medical and nonmedical specialties.

REFERENCES

American Board of Pediatrics, Inc. Foundations for Evaluating the Competency of Pediatricians. 1974. Chicago: American Board of Pediatrics, Inc.

APPENDIX

An example of the application of the tasks-by-abilities matrix to a clinical situation involving handicapping conditions

PROBLEM: A 26-year-old mother has a 2-year-old daughter who has Down's syndrome with acyanotic congenital heart disease and mild to moderate developmental delay. The mother is 12 weeks pregnant.

A-1 Attitudes — Data Gathering
  1. The resident asks what toys are available to the 2-year-old girl with Down's syndrome. (Curriculum Goal 1)
  2. The resident interacts directly with the child in the process of assessing her current adaptive developmental level. (Curriculum Goal 2)
  3. The resident obtains information about the mother's chromosome karyotype. (Curriculum Goal 4)
  4. The resident seeks evaluation of the 2-year-old girl's developmental level from at least one other professional (psychologist, special educator, speech and language clinician, or occupational therapist). (Curriculum Goal 6)
  5. The resident asks what the mother knows about tuition-free preschool programs for the handicapped in the child's community. (Curriculum Goal 12)
A-2 Attitudes — Assessment of Data
  1. The resident refers mother to state clinic for arranging chromo-

some analysis on learning that the family income is $8,000 per year. (Curriculum Goal 1)

2. The resident chooses to take extra time to explain to the mother the definition of "mild to moderate developmental delay" and the implications for future function on discovering that she believes it means that the child will never progress beyond the current 12- to 15-month developmental level. (Curriculum Goal 2)

3. The resident orders a repeat chromosome analysis on the mother and father when the 2-year-old's karyotype indicates 15/21 translocation and the mother's initial karyotype is reported as normal. (Curriculum Goal 4)

4. The resident calls the director of the child's preschool for a verbal report of the child's developmental level when receipt of the written report is delayed. (Curriculum Goal 6)

5. The resident reviews with the mother her rights to participate in the formulation of the individual educational plan for her child. (Curriculum Goal 12)

A-3 Attitudes — Management

1. The resident suggests a follow-up visit to discuss preschool adjustment and developmental progress within 3 months of initial visit. (Curriculum Goal 1)

2. The resident refers 2-year-old child for placement in an early intervention preschool program. (Curriculum Goal 2)

3. The resident discusses the relationship between amniocentesis and abortion with the mother regarding her current pregnancy. (Curriculum Goal 4)

4. The resident sends a copy of his follow-up developmental observations to the child's school and to the colleague who carried out the initial educational assessment. (Curriculum Goal 6)

5. The resident participates in a meeting at school scheduled to discuss the role of occupational therapy and speech therapy as supplements to the preschool classroom experience. (Curriculum Goal 7)

6. The resident offers to write the state legislature's Committee on Human Services in support of state funding for early education programs for Down's syndrome children. (Curriculum Goal 12)

B-1 Factual Knowledge — Data Gathering

1. The resident identifies how many months below the norm the 2-year-old is in each of a variety of typical developmental milestones. (Curriculum Goal 1)

2. The resident identifies the distinguishing clinical features of Trisomy 21. (Curriculum Goal 3)

3. The resident recognizes the chromosome karyotype of 46, XX, t(15;21). (Curriculum Goal 4)

4. The resident selects two appropriate assessment measures for evaluation of the 2-year-old's developmental level. (Curriculum Goal 5)

5. The resident identifies three appropriate assessment measures for the educational diagnostician's evaluation of the 2-year-old's developmental level. (Curriculum Goal 6)

6. The resident recognizes the appropriate admission diagnostic tests used by the early intervention preschool program for handicapped children. (Curriculum Goal 9)

7. The resident states the clinical symptoms and signs of the common forms of congenital heart disease associated with Down's syndrome. (Curriculum Goal 10)

8. The resident describes three studies documenting developmental differences between normal and Down's syndrome children. (Curriculum Goal 11)

9. The resident describes the criteria for state funding of developmental and medical diagnostic studies in the 2-year-old with Down's syndrome. (Curriculum Goal 12)

B-2 Factual Knowledge — Assessment of Data

1. The resident explains the factors leading to the difference in IQ between institutionalized and non-institutionalized children with Down's syndrome. (Curriculum Goals 1 and 11)

2. The resident states three theories explaining the increased frequency of Down's syndrome with advanced maternal age. (Curriculum Goal 3)

3. The resident states the risk that the fetus has Down's syndrome. (Curriculum Goal 3)

4. The resident states the possible reasons for discrepancies in developmental level of the 2-year-old noted on four different evaluation instruments. (Curriculum Goals 5 and 6)

5. The resident states the relationship between the early intervention preschool and the public school's special education department. (Curriculum Goals 9 and 12)

6. The resident states the prognosis of endocardial cushion defect. (Curriculum Goal 10)

B-3 Factual Knowledge — Management

1. The resident identifies age-appropriate behavior-management techniques for the mother to use while disciplining the 2-year-old. (Curriculum Goal 1)

2. The resident identifies the major curriculum areas for the 2-year-old's program this year and predicts those to be covered next year. (Curriculum Goals 3 and 7)

3. The resident describes when and how an amniocentesis will be performed. (Curriculum Goal 4)

4. The resident states the role that an occupational therapist and a speech therapist might play in the 2-year-old's program. (Curriculum Goal 6)
5. The resident describes the supplementary staff available at the preschool. (Curriculum Goal 9)
6. The resident states the criteria for cardiac catheterization and surgical repair of endocardial cushion defect. (Curriculum Goal 10)
7. The resident describes three studies documenting the effectiveness of early intervention programs for Down's syndrome children. (Curriculum Goal 11)
8. The resident describes how the public school will involve the mother in planning for future appropriate classroom placement. (Curriculum Goal 12)

C-1 Interpersonal Skills — Data Gathering
1. The resident looks at and responds to other professionals as they give reports of the 2-year-old's behavior at staffing conference. (Curriculum Goal 6)
2. The resident uses vocabulary that the mother is able to understand when obtaining perinatal and developmental history from her. (Curriculum Goal 8)
3. The resident speaks comfortingly to the 2-year-old as he examines her heart. (Curriculum Goal 10)

C-2 Interpersonal Skills — Assessment of Data
1. The resident listens to the prognosis of the 2-year-old as stated by other professionals at the staffing conference. (Curriculum Goal 6)
2. The resident discusses with the mother the prognosis of the 2-year-old's developmental progress in realistic but hopeful terms. (Curriculum Goal 8)
3. The resident discusses the child's heart lesion and its prognosis in terms the mother can understand. (Curriculum Goal 10)

C-3 Interpersonal Skills — Management
1. The resident explains the reasons for amniocentesis and the procedures the mother will go through to other professionals at the staffing conference. (Curriculum Goal 6)
2. The resident explains to the mother the advantages of a close relationship between the preschool and home experiences. (Curriculum Goals 7 and 8)
3. The resident discusses general health care needs (diet, exercise, sleep, play) with the mother. (Curriculum Goal 10)

D-1 Technical Skills — Data Gathering
1. The resident reliably carries out a brief standardized developmental assessment of the 2-year-old. (Curriculum Goal 5)

2. The resident accurately describes the 2-year-old's heart murmur. (Curriculum Goal 10)

D-2 Technical Skills — Assessment of Data

1. The resident accurately interprets the results of the standardized developmental assessment. (Curriculum Goal 5)

2. The resident accurately interprets the changes in the tympanic membranes of the 2-year-old. (Curriculum Goal 10)

D-3 Technical Skills — Management

1. The resident prescribes the appropriate medications for the 2-year-old's middle ear infection. (Curriculum Goal 10)

E-1 Clinical Judgment — Data Gathering

1. The resident seeks background data from each professional attending the staffing conference. (Curriculum Goal 6)

2. The resident arranges an interview alone with the mother upon finding that the 2-year-old's presence is distracting to her. (Curriculum Goal 8)

3. The resident sends for reports of all previous cardiac evaluations. (Curriculum Goal 10)

E-2 Clinical Judgment — Assessment of Data

1. The resident requests repeat testing when one team member reports developmental levels that are far out of line with other observers. (Curriculum Goal 6)

2. The resident asks to confer with both parents when he discovers the parents differ in their beliefs regarding abortion. (Curriculum Goal 8)

3. The resident orders appropriate further studies on discovering early signs of cardiac insufficiency. (Curriculum Goal 10)

E-3 Clinical Judgment — Management

1. The resident urges that a summary of all practical recommendations for management suggested by each professional at the staffing conference be made available and be interpreted to the mother and the preschool teacher. (Curriculum Goals 6 and 7)

2. The resident recommends to the mother that she visit the school and speak with the teacher at least biweekly and return for follow-up review of developmental progress at 2- or 3-month intervals. (Curriculum Goal 8)

3. The resident inquires about the professional training and developmental perspective of staff members at the preschool before referring the child there for placement. (Curriculum Goal 9)

4. The resident refers the child to a Pediatric Cardiology Clinic for definitive management of her congenital heart disease. (Curriculum Goal 10)

Author Index

Subject Index